List of Contents

Introduction: Unlocking the Power To Cure Diseases From Within

Welcome to the beginning of your powerful healing journey—a journey that will guide you towards a life of vibrant health and well-being. In these pages, we will embark on a voyage of self-discovery and empowerment, exploring the profound impact of mindful living and fasting in combatting diseases and nurturing a healthier, more resilient you.

Our modern world is a paradox. On one hand, we have unprecedented access to knowledge, technology, and conveniences that make life more comfortable than ever before. On the other, we find ourselves battling an alarming rise in chronic diseases, stress-related ailments, and a pervasive sense of disconnection from our own bodies.

It's as if we are living in two realms simultaneously: one where we have the tools for physical comfort and the other where our physical and mental well-being often hangs in the balance. It's clear that something is amiss, and many of us are seeking answers.

This book, "Combat Diseases with Mindful Living Techniques," will take you on a holistic journey toward health and vitality. We'll dive deep into the practice of mindful living—a practice rooted in ancient wisdom but adapted to the demands of our modern lives. We'll explore the art of fasting, a method that has been used for centuries to cleanse the body and foster healing. Together, we will uncover the incredible synergy between these two approaches and how they can help you achieve optimal health.

It all starts with an understanding of the profound mind-body connection. You see, your thoughts, emotions, and mental state are not separate from your physical health. They are deeply intertwined, affecting your well-being on a cellular level. Stress, anxiety, and negative thought patterns can manifest as physical symptoms, leading to a cascade of health issues.

Mindful living is not just a trendy concept; it is a science-backed approach to harmonizing the mind and body. By cultivating mindfulness—awareness of the present moment without judgment—you can reduce stress, enhance your immune system, and even influence your genetic expression. It's a power within you, waiting to be harnessed.

Before we delve into the practical aspects of mindful living and fasting, let's take a moment to appreciate the science that underpins these practices. These are not mere fads or quick fixes. They are grounded in rigorous research and have shown remarkable results.

Mindful living, as validated by countless studies, can improve mental health, reduce anxiety and depression, lower blood pressure, and enhance overall well-being. Its influence extends to physical health, as mindfulness practices have been linked to lower inflammation levels, better cardiovascular health, and even a reduction in chronic pain.

Fasting, too, is not a new-age trend. It has been an integral part of human history and is deeply rooted in our biology. Scientific research has revealed that fasting can trigger autophagy—a cellular cleaning process that removes damaged components and supports cellular health. It can also improve insulin sensitivity, aid in weight management, and reduce the risk of chronic diseases.

But here's where it gets exciting: when you combine mindful living with fasting, you unleash a potent force for healing and disease prevention. Mindful awareness enhances the fasting experience, making it more sustainable and impactful. And fasting, in turn, deepens your mindfulness practice, creating a harmonious cycle of physical and mental well-being.

As we journey through this book, you'll discover practical, actionable steps that will empower you to incorporate mindful living and fasting into your daily life. We won't just explore the theory; we'll dive into real-life applications. You'll learn how to meditate effectively, practice mindful eating, and create a mindful environment that nurtures your well-being.

Fasting will no longer be a mysterious concept but a deliberate choice to support your health. We'll explore various fasting methods and provide guidance on how to choose the one that aligns with your goals and lifestyle. You'll find strategies for preparing for a fast, breaking it safely, and navigating potential challenges along the way.

But remember, this isn't a one-size-fits-all journey. Your path to health is uniquely yours. We'll help you personalize your approach, taking into account your individual needs and circumstances.

In the chapters that follow, we will explore the mind-body connection, delve into the science of mindful living and fasting, and provide you with practical, actionable steps to start your transformative journey. Together, we will navigate the challenges, celebrate the successes, and uncover the incredible potential that resides within you.

So, let's prepare on this adventure of self-discovery, healing, and empowerment. Your health, your happiness, and your future await. It's time to take the first step towards a life of vibrant well-being.

Chapter 1: Understanding Mindful Living for Disease Prevention

1.1 What is Mindful Living?

Welcome to the journey of understanding mindful living and how it can be your most potent tool in the battle against diseases. In this chapter, we'll delve deep into what mindful living truly means, uncovering its profound principles, exploring the intricate mind-body connection, and unveiling how mindfulness becomes the guardian of our well-being.

Definition and Principles of Mindful Living

Mindful living is more than just a trendy words; it's a way of life that has the potential to transform every facet of your existence. At its core, mindful living is about being fully present, consciously engaged, and acutely aware of every moment. It's the art of paying attention to your thoughts, emotions, sensations, and surroundings without judgment.

Imagine a typical day. How often do you find yourself lost in thought, ruminating over the past, or worrying about the future, completely detached from the present moment? Mindful living is the antidote to this mental drift. It's the practice of anchoring yourself in the here and now, cultivating an unwavering focus on whatever you're doing, be it eating, walking, or simply breathing.

The principles of mindful living are beautifully simple:

1. Non-Judgmental Awareness: This means observing your thoughts and feelings without criticizing or labeling them as good or bad. It's about acknowledging your inner experiences with compassion and detachment.

2. Present-Moment Focus: Mindful living encourages you to shift your attention from dwelling on the past or worrying about the future to fully engaging in what's happening right now. This empowers you to savor the richness of each moment.

3. Acceptance: Acceptance is a cornerstone of mindfulness. It involves recognizing and embracing your current reality, whether it's pleasant or challenging, without attempting to change it. Through acceptance, you learn to respond to life's ups and downs with equanimity.

4. Openness: Being open means approaching life with a curious, receptive attitude. It's about letting go of preconceived notions and embracing novelty and unpredictability.

5. Engagement: Mindful living invites you to wholeheartedly engage in whatever you're doing, whether it's a mundane task or a joyful experience. It's about infusing your actions with intention and presence.

The Mind-Body Connection and Its Impact on Health
Now, let's explore the intriguing mind-body connection. Your mind and body are not isolated entities; they are deeply intertwined, constantly communicating with each

other. What happens in your mind can profoundly influence your physical health.

Consider stress, for instance. When you're under chronic stress, your mind perceives threats everywhere, releasing stress hormones like cortisol and adrenaline. These hormones, in turn, trigger a cascade of physical responses in your body, raising blood pressure, compromising the immune system, and increasing inflammation. Over time, this chronic stress can contribute to the development of various diseases, including cardiovascular issues, digestive disorders, and even mental health challenges like anxiety and depression.

On the flip side, when you embrace mindful living, you step onto a path of stress reduction. By being present and managing your responses to stressors, you signal to your body that it's safe to relax. This prompts the release of calming hormones like oxytocin and endorphins, promoting physical relaxation, immune system support, and enhanced overall well-being.

Furthermore, mindfulness can positively impact your immune system. Studies have shown that mindfulness practices can increase the production of antibodies and enhance the body's ability to fight off infections. It's as if your mind is sending signals to your immune system, saying, "I'm aware, I'm at ease, and I'm ready to defend."

The impact of mindfulness extends to pain management as well. When you're mindful, you can alter your perception of pain. It doesn't eliminate pain, but it changes your relationship with it. By observing pain with a non-judgmental attitude, you can reduce the suffering associated with it.

So, the mind-body connection is a powerful ally in disease prevention. When you practice mindful living, you're not just nurturing your mind; you're also nurturing your body and fortifying it against the perils of stress and illness.

The Role of Mindfulness in Disease Prevention
Now, let's talk about the star of the show: mindfulness in disease prevention. Mindfulness isn't a magical potion that guarantees immunity to all ailments, but it is a potent shield that fortifies your defenses and boosts your resilience.

Here's how mindfulness contributes to disease prevention:

1. Stress Reduction: We've already touched upon this, but it's worth emphasizing how critical stress reduction is. Chronic stress is a significant contributor to numerous diseases, from hypertension to diabetes. By practicing mindfulness, you reduce stress's harmful impact on your body.

2. Immune System Support: Mindfulness enhances immune function, making your body better equipped to fend off infections and diseases.

3. Better Decision-Making: Mindful living sharpens your decision-making abilities. When you're mindful, you're less likely to engage in impulsive, unhealthy behaviors like overeating, smoking, or excessive drinking.

4. Healthy Eating Habits: Mindful eating, a subset of mindful living, can transform your relationship with food. By paying close attention to the sensations of hunger and fullness, as well as the flavors and textures of your meals, you're more likely to make nutritious choices.

5. Emotional Well-being: Many diseases have psychological components, and mindfulness can be a powerful tool in managing them. Whether it's anxiety, depression, or chronic pain, mindfulness can help you cope more effectively.

6. Preventing Lifestyle-Related Diseases: Diseases like type 2 diabetes, obesity, and heart disease are often linked to lifestyle factors. Mindful living encourages healthier choices and habits, reducing the risk of these conditions.

Mindfulness acts as your proactive partner in the journey of disease prevention. It equips you with the tools to make informed, health-conscious decisions and respond to life's challenges with resilience and grace. Mindful living is a practice, a journey, and a lifelong commitment. It's not about achieving perfection but about embracing imperfection with kindness and awareness.

1.2 Mindfulness Practices

In the cacophony of modern life, where smartphones buzz incessantly and schedules stretch us to our limits, it's easy to lose touch with ourselves. Amid the hustle and bustle, the art of mindful living emerges as a beacon of hope, offering not just respite but also a powerful tool for combating diseases and fostering overall well-being. In this subchapter, we'll delve into mindfulness practices - a cornerstone of mindful living - and explore their profound impact on our health and disease prevention.

Meditation and Its Health Benefits

Let's begin our journey into the realm of mindfulness with meditation, a practice that has stood the test of time as a means to center the mind and cultivate a state of profound awareness. While it might conjure images of yogis sitting cross-legged atop misty mountain peaks, meditation is a practice accessible to anyone, anywhere.

The scientific community has been fervently studying meditation, and their findings have been nothing short of remarkable. Regular meditation not only alters the brain's structure but also enhances its function. The gray matter in the brain's amygdala, associated with stress and fear, tends to shrink with consistent meditation, while the prefrontal cortex, responsible for decision-making and emotional regulation, expands. This translates to better stress management, improved emotional resilience, and a heightened ability to focus.

Yes, you read that right – mindfulness meditation can actually bolster your immune system. Studies have shown that regular meditation enhances the production of antibodies and activates natural killer cells, making your body more adept at warding off infections. The simple act of sitting in stillness, focusing on your breath, and being present has the power to boost your body's natural defenses.

Embarking on a meditation journey might seem daunting, but it's simpler than you think. Start with just a few minutes each day. Find a quiet spot, sit comfortably, close your eyes, and focus on your breath. When your mind inevitably drifts, gently guide it back to your breath. Over time, you'll find yourself experiencing moments of profound clarity and inner peace that will seep into your daily life, making you more resilient in the face of stress and disease.

Mindful Eating and Its Impact on Nutrition
Now, let's turn our attention to another facet of mindfulness - mindful eating. In a world where fast food is the norm and mealtime is often a rushed affair, this practice invites us to slow down, savor each bite, and reconnect with our bodies.

Mindful eating encourages you to savor your food slowly, paying attention to every texture, flavor, and aroma. This heightened awareness not only deepens your appreciation for your meals but also helps prevent overeating. You'll find that you can enjoy your favorite dishes without needing to consume as much because you're fully present and satisfied with each bite.

Mindful eating is not just about savoring what's on your plate; it's also about making conscious choices. It empowers you to listen to your body's cues and make decisions based on hunger and nourishment rather than emotional impulses. You become attuned to your body's signals, allowing you to differentiate between genuine hunger and stress-induced cravings.

Research has shown that mindful eating can have a profound impact on nutrition and, by extension, disease prevention. It can lead to better weight management, improved blood sugar control, and even a reduced risk of heart disease. By paying attention to the quality and quantity of your food, you can make choices that support your health and vitality.

Incorporating Mindfulness into Daily Routines
Lastly, let's explore how you can weave mindfulness into the tapestry of your daily life. While meditation and mindful eating are intentional practices, mindfulness in your daily routines is about infusing every moment with conscious awareness.

1: Mindful Breathing Throughout the Day

One of the simplest ways to bring mindfulness into your daily life is through your breath. No matter where you are or what you're doing, you can always return to your breath as an anchor to the present moment. Take a few deep breaths, focusing your attention on the sensation of the breath entering and leaving your body. This quick exercise can instantly calm your mind and reduce stress.

2: Mindful Walking and Movement

Walking is an activity we do every day, yet it often goes unnoticed. Mindful walking involves paying attention to each step, the feeling of your feet on the ground, and the rhythm of your stride. It's a meditation in motion that can be practiced while strolling through a park, walking to work, or even while doing chores. By grounding yourself in the act of walking, you invite mindfulness into your daily routine.

3: Mindful Moments of Pause

Throughout your day, make it a habit to pause and take a mindful moment. This can be as simple as pausing before a meeting to take a few breaths or savoring a moment of stillness before diving into a task. These mindful pauses serve as mini-resets, helping you stay centered and focused amid life's demands.

Incorporating mindfulness into your daily routines doesn't require extra time; it's about infusing intention and awareness into the activities you're already engaged in. By doing so, you'll find yourself more grounded, less stressed, and better equipped to prevent disease by nurturing your overall well-being. These practices are your keys to unlocking the transformative power of mindful living and disease prevention. As you continue practice it, you'll discover how these practices synergize with fasting and other mindful living techniques to create a holistic approach to your health and well-being.

1.3 Mindful Living and Disease Prevention

In the bustling rhythm of modern life, the pursuit of health and happiness can often feel like an elusive dream. We find ourselves juggling responsibilities, racing against the clock, and navigating a sea of distractions. Yet, in the midst of this chaos, there exists a powerful and transformative practice that has the potential to change the course of our lives – mindful living.

How Mindful Living Can Reduce Diseases

Imagine a world where the burden of diseases like heart disease, diabetes, and stress-related disorders is significantly lighter. In this world, individuals have unlocked the incredible potential of their own minds to promote health and ward off the looming shadows of illness. This isn't the stuff of science fiction; it's the reality that mindful living can bring into your life.

Mindful living, at its core, is about cultivating an unwavering awareness of the present moment. It's about being fully engaged with the here and now, rather than dwelling in the past or constantly worrying about the future. While this may sound deceptively simple, its effects on your health can be profound.

When you live mindfully, you begin to notice the subtleties of your body and mind. You become attuned to the signals they send you. You recognize the early whispers of stress, tension, or discomfort that, left unchecked, could manifest as serious health issues down the road.

Mindful living encourages a proactive approach to health. Instead of waiting for symptoms to escalate or diseases to take root, you're actively involved in your own well-being. By paying attention to the present moment, you're better equipped to identify the factors contributing to your health, such as dietary choices, stress levels, and sleep patterns.

Consider the impact of stress, for example. Chronic stress is a silent predator that can wreak havoc on your health. It's linked to a wide array of ailments, from hypertension to gastrointestinal disorders. But when you live mindfully, you're armed with a powerful antidote against stress – awareness.

You notice the tension in your shoulders as you sit at your desk, the racing thoughts that accompany an impending deadline, or the shallow breaths you take during a hectic day. This heightened awareness gives you the choice to respond differently. You can choose to step away from your desk for a few minutes, take deep, calming breaths, or engage in a brief mindfulness meditation. These actions, seemingly small, can prevent stress from snowballing into a full-blown health crisis.

Mindfulness for Better Sleep and Immunity
The relationship between mindfulness and sleep is a profound one. In a world where sleep disorders are increasingly common, and insomnia is a frequent visitor to our bedrooms, the gift of restful, restorative sleep is something many of us yearn for. Yet, often, the more we chase sleep, the more elusive it becomes.

Mindful living extends its gentle hand here as well. It offers a sanctuary for your racing mind, a refuge from the endless to-do lists and worries that often flood your thoughts as you lay in bed. When you practice mindfulness, you learn to let go of the mental chatter that keeps you awake at night.

One of the key tenets of mindful living is the practice of mindful breathing. It's a simple technique that can be applied to almost any aspect of your life, including your sleep. As you lay in bed, focus your attention on your breath. Feel the rise and fall of your chest, the cool air as you inhale and the warm air as you exhale. Your mind may wander, but gently guide it back to your breath. This repetitive act of bringing your awareness back to the present moment has a calming effect that can usher you into a peaceful slumber.

Moreover, practicing mindfulness during the day can reduce the accumulation of stress that might otherwise disrupt your sleep. Remember, sleep and immunity are closely linked. When you don't get enough sleep, your immune system's defenses weaken, leaving you vulnerable to infections and illnesses. By integrating mindfulness into your daily routine, you're not only improving the quality of your sleep but also bolstering your body's ability to fend off diseases.

Mindful Communication and Healthier Relationships

Our journey into mindful living wouldn't be complete without exploring its impact on our relationships. In a world that often pushes us toward constant busyness and superficial connections, mindful communication offers a profound antidote.

Mindful communication isn't just about being a better listener or articulating your thoughts more clearly. It's about fostering genuine connections, empathy, and compassion. These qualities are like healing balms for the wounds that relationships can sometimes inflict.

When you engage in mindful communication, you're fully present with the person you're talking to. You're not distracted by your phone, your thoughts, or your own agenda. You're there, in the moment, listening not just with your ears but with your heart. This kind of presence can mend broken bonds and create deeper, more meaningful connections.

In the realm of health, the benefits of healthier relationships are manifold. Consider the impact of stress on your well-being. Stress often finds its way into our lives through our interactions with others – be it a difficult colleague, a strained family relationship, or an unresolved conflict with a friend. When you practice mindful communication, you're better equipped to navigate these challenges.

You're less likely to react impulsively or say hurtful things in the heat of the moment. Instead, you respond thoughtfully, with empathy and understanding. This not only diffuses tense situations but also protects your own health from the damaging effects of chronic stress.

Mindful living and mindful communication work in tandem to create a ripple effect of wellness. As you improve your own well-being through mindfulness, you naturally become a source of positivity and support for those around you. Your healthier habits and emotional resilience can inspire others to embark on their own journeys toward better health.

We've seen how mindfulness can reduce diseases by fostering awareness of your body and mind, improving sleep and immunity, and enhancing your communication and relationships. But this is just the beginning. The journey of mindful living is a deeply personal one, and its potential to transform your life is limitless.

Chapter 2: The Power of Fasting for Health and Healing

2.1 Exploring Different Fasting Methods

In our journey towards combating diseases and achieving optimal health through mindful living, fasting emerges as a powerful ally. Fasting has been practiced for centuries, not just as a means to satisfy spiritual or cultural traditions but also as a remarkable tool for health and healing. In this chapter, we'll delve into the world of fasting, explore different fasting methods, and help you discover the fasting approach that suits you best.

Intermittent Fasting and Its Variations

Intermittent fasting (IF) is like the Swiss Army knife of fasting methods – versatile, adaptable, and highly effective. At its core, intermittent fasting involves cycling between periods of eating and fasting. What sets IF apart is its flexibility. It allows you to choose a fasting window that aligns with your lifestyle and preferences.

1: The 16/8 Method

 - The 16/8 method is a popular IF variation. It entails fasting for 16 hours and restricting eating to an 8-hour window. Most people find it practical to skip breakfast and consume their first meal around noon, then conclude their eating window by 8 PM.

 - This approach capitalizes on the overnight fasting period when the body taps into stored energy reserves, helping to regulate blood sugar levels and enhance fat metabolism. It's a great starting point for those new to fasting.

2: The 5:2 Method

 - For those who prefer a more intermittent approach, the 5:2 method might be appealing. With this variation, you eat normally for five days of the week and restrict calorie intake to around 500-600 calories on the remaining two non-consecutive days.

 - This method allows for greater dietary freedom on regular days while still reaping the benefits of intermittent fasting, such as improved insulin sensitivity and weight management.

3: Eat-Stop-Eat

 - Eat-Stop-Eat is a straightforward approach involving a full 24-hour fast once or twice a week. You would have dinner, fast for 24 hours, and then resume eating with dinner the following day.

 - While this method requires a bit more discipline, it provides extended periods for your body to engage in cellular repair and detoxification, promoting overall health and longevity.

Extended Fasts and Their Potential Benefits
Extended fasts push the boundaries of fasting duration, and
they are often seen as a deeper dive into the world of
fasting. These fasts typically last from 48 hours to several
days or even weeks. While they may sound challenging, the
rewards can be profound.

1: The 48-Hour Fast

 - A 48-hour fast is exactly what it sounds like: abstaining
from food for two full days. It's an excellent way to reset
your metabolism, improve insulin sensitivity, and initiate
the body's repair processes.

 - During this fast, your body switches to burning stored fat
for energy, which can lead to weight loss and
improvements in various health markers.

2: The 3-Day Water Fast

 - The 3-day water fast is a more extended variation that
involves consuming only water for three consecutive days.
This method takes you deeper into the realms of autophagy,
the body's natural process of self-cleaning and repair.

 - While it may sound intimidating, many people find it
easier than expected, thanks to the body's adaptive response
to fasting. It's crucial to approach this fast with adequate
preparation and a focus on hydration.

3: Extended Fasts and Healing

 - Extended fasts, beyond three days, have been associated with remarkable health benefits. They can be a powerful tool in combating chronic diseases, reducing inflammation, and promoting cellular regeneration.

 - These longer fasts should be undertaken with caution and ideally under the guidance of a healthcare professional. They require careful planning and a gradual approach, especially if you're new to fasting.

Choosing the Right Fasting Method for You
The beauty of fasting is that it's not a one-size-fits-all approach. There's a fasting method to suit every individual, and the key lies in finding the one that aligns with your goals, preferences, and lifestyle.

1: Self-Discovery Through Experimentation

 - Start by experimenting with different fasting methods and observing how your body responds. Some people may thrive on intermittent fasting, while others may find extended fasts more suitable.

 - Keep a journal to track your energy levels, mood, and overall well-being during fasting periods. This self-awareness will guide you in choosing the right fasting approach.

2: Consider Your Goals

  - What are your health and wellness goals? Are you looking to lose weight, improve insulin sensitivity, or target a specific health condition? Your goals can influence the fasting method that suits you best.

  - For example, if your primary goal is weight loss, intermittent fasting may be an excellent starting point. On the other hand, if you're aiming for deep cellular healing, you might explore extended fasts under professional supervision.

3: Listen to Your Body

  - Your body is a wise and intuitive guide. Pay attention to hunger cues, energy levels, and how you feel during fasting and eating periods. Don't force a fasting method that doesn't align with your body's signals.

  - If a particular fasting regimen feels unsustainable or overly challenging, it's perfectly okay to adapt and try a different approach. The key is to find a sustainable and enjoyable fasting practice.

Fasting is a remarkable tool for health and healing, offering a spectrum of methods that can be tailored to your unique needs. Whether you opt for intermittent fasting to kickstart your journey or venture into the depths of extended fasts, remember that fasting is a journey of self-discovery and empowerment. It's about nourishing not just your body but also your mind and spirit, ultimately leading you towards a healthier and more vibrant life.

2.2 Fasting and Cellular Health

In our fast-paced world, where instant gratification is the norm, the idea of willingly abstaining from food may seem counterintuitive. Yet, fasting, when approached mindfully and strategically, holds profound potential for healing and rejuvenation at the cellular level. In this subchapter, we'll dive deep into the fascinating realm of fasting and cellular health, exploring how it triggers autophagy, promotes metabolic health, and serves as a powerful tool for reducing inflammation.

Autophagy and Cellular Repair during Fasting

Imagine your body as a bustling city, with cells serving as its dedicated workers. Each cell has its tasks, from producing energy to fighting off invaders. But just like a city, our cells generate waste. Autophagy, a term derived from the Greek words "auto" (self) and "phagein" (to eat), is the cellular waste disposal system—a critical process that becomes supercharged during fasting.

During fasting, especially prolonged or intermittent fasting, your body senses the scarcity of incoming nutrients. To adapt, it shifts into a mode that prioritizes survival and efficient resource utilization. This is where autophagy comes into play. It's as if your cells start cleaning house, breaking down and recycling damaged proteins, organelles, and other cellular components.

Think of it like renovating an old building. Autophagy removes the worn-out bricks, repairs the foundation, and replaces outdated systems. This cellular cleanup has profound implications for your health. It helps prevent the accumulation of damaged molecules and dysfunctional cellular components, reducing the risk of various diseases, including cancer and neurodegenerative disorders.

But how can you harness the power of autophagy through fasting in a practical way? Here's an actionable step:

Actionable Step 1: Intermittent Fasting for Cellular Cleanup

- Start with a 12-hour fast: If you're new to fasting, begin by extending your overnight fast. Finish dinner at 7 pm and delay breakfast until 7 am the next day. This simple 12-hour fast helps your body dip its toes into autophagy.

- Gradually increase the fasting window: As you become comfortable with a 12-hour fast, gradually extend it to 14, 16, or even 18 hours. These longer fasting periods enhance autophagy and provide more significant cellular repair benefits.

- Stay hydrated: During your fasting window, drink plenty of water, herbal tea, or black coffee (without added sugar or cream). Staying hydrated supports the cleansing process.

Fasting for Metabolic Health and Weight Management

Fasting isn't just about emptying the trash within your cells; it's also about recalibrating your metabolism. In our modern world, where overconsumption is rampant, our bodies often struggle with excess calories and insulin resistance, leading to obesity and metabolic disorders. Fasting offers a reset button for your metabolism.

When you fast, especially during extended fasts, your insulin levels drop, allowing your body to tap into its fat stores for energy. This promotes weight loss and fat burning. But fasting goes beyond weight management; it helps regulate blood sugar levels, reduce insulin resistance, and even lower the risk of type 2 diabetes.

Actionable Step 2: Intermittent Fasting for Metabolic Health

- Start with a 16/8 schedule: Adopt the 16/8 intermittent fasting method, where you fast for 16 hours and have an 8-hour eating window. For instance, eat between 12 pm and 8 pm, and fast from 8 pm to 12 pm the next day.

- Focus on whole foods: During your eating window, prioritize nutrient-dense, whole foods like vegetables, lean proteins, and healthy fats. Avoid processed foods and excessive sugar to optimize metabolic health.

- Monitor your progress: Keep a journal to track your fasting hours, meals, and how you feel. Pay attention to changes in your energy levels, weight, and blood sugar. This self-awareness will guide your fasting journey.

Fasting as a Tool for Reducing Inflammation
Chronic inflammation is the silent villain behind many chronic diseases. It's like a fire burning within your body, causing damage to tissues and organs over time. Fasting acts as a natural extinguisher, dampening this inflammatory fire and reducing the risk of inflammatory-related conditions, such as heart disease, arthritis, and autoimmune disorders.

During fasting, your body switches gears from growth mode to repair mode. It downregulates inflammatory pathways and activates processes that repair tissues and reduce inflammation. This anti-inflammatory effect is partly due to the reduction in circulating insulin levels and the secretion of anti-inflammatory molecules during fasting.

Actionable Step 3: Intermittent Fasting for Inflammation Control

- Choose whole, anti-inflammatory foods: When you break your fast, focus on foods known for their anti-inflammatory properties. Include berries, fatty fish rich in omega-3s, turmeric, and leafy greens in your meals.

- Combine fasting with mindfulness: Incorporate mindfulness practices like meditation or deep breathing into your daily routine. Stress reduction through mindfulness complements fasting's anti-inflammatory benefits.

- Gradually increase fasting duration: As your body adapts, consider longer fasting periods (e.g., 24-hour fasts) intermittently to enhance the anti-inflammatory effects.

Fasting is a powerful tool for enhancing cellular health, improving metabolic function, and reducing inflammation. By incorporating intermittent fasting into your lifestyle and understanding its mechanisms, you can embark on a journey of healing and rejuvenation at the cellular level. Remember, your body has an innate ability to heal itself when given the right conditions, and fasting, approached mindfully, provides those conditions.

2.3 Safe and Effective Fasting Practices

In the previous subchapters, we've explored the various types of fasting and the incredible impact it can have on your health and healing journey. Now, we dive deeper into the practical aspects of fasting, ensuring that you embark on this powerful journey safely and effectively.

Fasting isn't just about abstaining from food; it's a conscious decision to give your body a break, allowing it to rejuvenate and heal. To make the most of fasting, you must be prepared, approach it mindfully, and be aware of potential risks and precautions.

Preparing for a Fast and Breaking It Safely

Before you start any fasting regimen, preparation is key. It's like getting ready for a marathon; you wouldn't just jump into it without training. Here's how to prepare for a fast:

1. Assess Your Health: Consult with a healthcare professional, especially if you have underlying health issues. Fasting might not be suitable for everyone, so it's essential to get personalized guidance.

2. Choose the Right Fast: Select the fasting method that aligns with your goals and abilities. If you're new to fasting, start with shorter, less restrictive fasts like intermittent fasting before attempting extended fasts.

3. Mindful Transition: Gradually reduce your food intake leading up to the fast. This eases your body into the process and minimizes the shock of suddenly not eating.

4. Stay Hydrated: Proper hydration is crucial. Drink plenty of water in the days leading up to your fast, and consider adding electrolytes or herbal teas for extra support.

5. Plan Your Meals: If you're practicing intermittent fasting, plan your meals during your eating window thoughtfully. Focus on nutrient-dense foods to ensure you're getting essential vitamins and minerals.

Now, let's talk about how to break your fast safely, which is just as important as the fast itself:

1. Start Slowly: After a prolonged fast, your digestive system needs time to adapt. Begin with small, easily digestible foods like fruit or a small salad.

2. Chew Mindfully: Pay attention to your chewing. Chewing thoroughly aids digestion and prevents discomfort.

3. Avoid Heavy Meals: Steer clear of heavy, greasy, or spicy foods immediately after fasting. Opt for lean proteins, vegetables, and whole grains.

4. Stay Hydrated: Rehydrate with water, herbal teas, or broths. Avoid sugary drinks or caffeine in the initial hours.

5. Listen to Your Body: Everyone's body responds differently. If you experience discomfort or digestive issues, don't be discouraged. It's a learning process, and your body will adapt over time.

Combining Mindful Living with Fasting for Optimal Results

Fasting isn't just about abstaining from food; it's a holistic approach that integrates seamlessly with mindful living practices. When you marry fasting with mindfulness, you create a powerful synergy for healing and well-being. Here's how to combine them effectively:

1. Mindful Eating: When you do eat, do it mindfully. Pay attention to every bite, savoring the flavors and textures. Avoid distractions like TV or smartphones during meals.

2. Emotional Awareness: Recognize your emotional triggers for eating. Are you eating out of stress, boredom, or genuine hunger? Mindfulness helps you differentiate and make healthier choices.

3. Stress Management: Stress can impact fasting negatively. Incorporate stress-reduction techniques like meditation, deep breathing, or yoga into your daily routine to support your fasting journey.

4. Listen to Your Body: Mindful living encourages you to listen to your body's signals. If you're fasting and your body says it needs nourishment, it's okay to break the fast mindfully and try again later.

Potential Risks and Precautions During Fasting
While fasting can bring numerous health benefits, it's not without its risks, especially if not done mindfully or inappropriately. Here are some potential risks and precautions to be aware of:

1. Nutrient Deficiency: Extended fasts can lead to nutrient deficiencies if not properly planned. Ensure you're getting essential vitamins and minerals through supplementation or thoughtful food choices during eating windows.

2. Dehydration: It's easy to underestimate your fluid needs during fasting. Dehydration can occur, so monitor your water intake and consider electrolyte supplements, especially during prolonged fasts.

3. Low Blood Sugar: Fasting can lead to low blood sugar (hypoglycemia), which can cause dizziness or fainting. If you experience these symptoms, break your fast with a small, easily digestible snack.

4. Eating Disorders: Fasting should not be a cover for disordered eating patterns. If you have a history of eating disorders, consult a healthcare professional before attempting any form of fasting.

5. Medication Interactions: Fasting may affect how medications are absorbed or metabolized. Consult with your healthcare provider to adjust medication schedules if necessary.

6. Pregnancy and Nursing: Fasting during pregnancy or while nursing can impact both you and your child's health. It's generally not recommended without medical supervision.

7. Individual Variation: Keep in mind that everyone's body responds differently to fasting. What works for one person may not work for another. Pay attention to how your body reacts and adapt your fasting regimen accordingly.

Fasting can be a powerful tool for health and healing when approached with care and mindfulness. Preparing for a fast, breaking it safely, combining it with mindful living, and being aware of potential risks are all vital aspects of a successful fasting journey. Remember, your health is a lifelong journey, and fasting can be one of the many tools in your wellness toolkit when used wisely and mindfully.

Chapter 3: The Mind-Body Connection in Disease Prevention

3.1 Psychoneuroimmunology and Health

In the realm of holistic health and well-being, the mind-body connection is a profound and often underappreciated force. It's a bridge that links our emotions, thoughts, and mental state to the intricate workings of our immune system. In this subchapter, we're about to dig deeper the field of psychoneuroimmunology—a mouthful of a term that simply means understanding how our emotions impact our immunity.

Understanding the Link Between Emotions and the Immune System

Let's begin by acknowledging a simple truth: our emotions aren't confined to our minds alone. They ripple through our entire being, influencing every nook and cranny of our physical and mental landscape. When it comes to our immune system, these emotions play a pivotal role.

Imagine a scenario where you've had a particularly stressful day at work. Deadlines loom, emails flood your inbox, and your patience wears thin. In this state, your body's stress response kicks into high gear. Hormones like cortisol flood your bloodstream, preparing you for the proverbial fight-or-flight response. It's an ancient survival mechanism, but in today's world, it often translates into chronic stress.

Now, here's the kicker: chronic stress isn't just a mental burden; it's a physical one too. Prolonged stress weakens our immune system's defenses. It's as if our body shifts resources away from immune function to deal with the perceived threat. This can leave us more susceptible to infections, allergies, and even chronic diseases.

Conversely, positive emotions like happiness, love, and gratitude have been shown to enhance our immune function. They're like a soothing balm for our body's defenses, bolstering our ability to fend off illnesses. It's not merely anecdotal; scientific studies have uncovered the tangible benefits of positive emotions on health.

So, the first actionable step here is clear: prioritize your emotional well-being. Understand that your emotions are not just fleeting thoughts; they are potent forces shaping your physical health. Cultivate positivity, practice gratitude, and seek moments of joy—it's not just a matter of feeling good; it's a matter of feeling well.

Stress Reduction for Immune System Resilience
Now that we've grasped the pivotal role of emotions, let's delve deeper into the world of stress—a ubiquitous companion in our modern lives. Stress is a double-edged sword. In acute situations, it can sharpen our focus and prepare us for action. But when chronic, it becomes a silent saboteur of our well-being.

As we've already touched upon, chronic stress can significantly compromise our immune system. It's like a constant drumbeat, wearing down our body's defenses over time. So, the second actionable step is to manage and mitigate stress effectively.

One of the most powerful tools in this regard is mindfulness. Mindfulness is not some esoteric practice reserved for meditation gurus atop distant mountains. It's a down-to-earth, practical approach to stress management that anyone can adopt.

Mindfulness involves paying attention to the present moment without judgment. It's about being fully present, whether you're sipping your morning coffee, walking in the park, or even navigating a hectic workday. It's the antidote to the chronic mental chatter and worries that perpetuate stress.

When we practice mindfulness, we create a buffer against stress. We become better equipped to respond calmly to life's challenges, rather than reacting with anxiety or anger. This, in turn, allows our immune system to operate optimally.

So, here's your actionable step number two: embrace mindfulness. Start with just a few minutes a day. Close your eyes, take a deep breath, and immerse yourself in the sensations of the present moment. Over time, this practice can become a powerful shield against the corrosive effects of stress on your immune system.

Mindfulness Practices to Boost Immunity
Now, let's explore the practical side of incorporating mindfulness into your life to boost immunity. Mindfulness

isn't a one-size-fits-all practice; it comes in various forms, and you can tailor it to suit your preferences and lifestyle.

1. Meditation for Immune Enhancement: Meditation isn't just about finding inner peace; it's also a potent immune booster. Regular meditation has been linked to increased production of antibodies, which play a crucial role in defending against pathogens. Set aside a few minutes each day to meditate, focusing on your breath or a specific mantra. Over time, you'll notice a greater sense of calm and, hopefully, improved immunity.

2. Mindful Eating for Nourishment: Your diet has a profound impact on your immune system. Practicing mindful eating involves savoring each bite, paying attention to flavors and textures, and eating without distractions. By being present during meals, you're more likely to make nourishing food choices that support your immune health. So, put away the screens and relish your meals consciously.

3. Movement as Mindfulness: Exercise doesn't have to be a mindless routine; it can be a mindfulness practice in itself. Whether it's yoga, tai chi, or simply a mindful walk in nature, physical activity can be an opportunity to anchor yourself in the present moment. These practices not only reduce stress but also promote immune resilience.

4. Mindful Breathing for Calm: Your breath is a constant anchor to the present moment. When stress creeps in, take a moment to pause and breathe deeply. Inhale slowly through your nose, feeling the air fill your lungs, and exhale through your mouth, letting go of tension. Repeat this

several times to create a sense of calm and reinforce your immune system.

By incorporating these mindfulness practices into your daily life, you're not only nurturing your emotional well-being but also fostering a resilient immune system. This of course isn't a one-time fix; it's a journey of self-care and self-discovery that can lead to lasting health benefits.

3.2 Mindfulness and Pain Management

Pain is a universal experience; it's an alarm system designed to protect us from harm. However, when pain becomes chronic, it can significantly disrupt our lives and overall well-being. In this subchapter, we'll explore the powerful role of mindfulness in managing and alleviating chronic pain. Through mindful approaches to pain relief, mind-body techniques for reducing pain perception, and the integration of mindfulness into complementary therapies, you'll discover practical strategies that can help you regain control over your life and find relief from persistent pain.

Mindful Approaches to Chronic Pain Relief

Chronic pain often feels like an uninvited guest that has overstayed its welcome. It can manifest in various forms – from backaches and migraines to conditions like fibromyalgia or arthritis. The first step in managing chronic pain through mindfulness is developing an acute awareness of it. Here's how:

1. Acknowledge the Pain: Begin by acknowledging your pain without judgment. Mindfulness invites you to observe your pain without categorizing it as good or bad. When you acknowledge your pain, you give yourself permission to experience it fully.

2. Breathe Through It: Breathing mindfully can be a game-changer. When pain flares up, focus on your breath. Inhale deeply and exhale slowly. This simple act can help relax your body and reduce the tension that often accompanies pain.

3. Body Scan Meditation: Regular body scan meditations can help you identify areas of tension and pain. Start at the top of your head and slowly scan down through your body, paying attention to any sensations you encounter. By doing this regularly, you can pinpoint areas that need attention.

4. Cultivate Patience: Healing takes time. Be patient with yourself. Mindfulness encourages you to embrace your pain as part of your experience and recognize that it won't last forever. This perspective shift can ease the emotional burden of chronic pain.

Mind-Body Techniques for Reducing Pain Perception

Our perception of pain is not solely determined by physical factors; our mental and emotional states play a significant role. Mind-body techniques can help alter our perception of pain, making it more manageable. Here's how you can apply these techniques:

1. Visualization: Close your eyes and visualize a place where you feel safe and relaxed. Imagine yourself there, away from the pain. This practice can reduce the intensity of pain signals sent to your brain.

2. Deep Relaxation: Progressive muscle relaxation and deep relaxation exercises can alleviate muscle tension and reduce pain. By consciously relaxing each muscle group, you can ease physical discomfort.

3. Mindful Distraction: Engaging in activities that require your full attention, such as puzzles or hobbies, can temporarily divert your focus from pain. The more absorbed you become in an activity, the less you may notice the pain.

4. Emotional Processing: Sometimes, pain is intertwined with unresolved emotions. Mindfulness encourages you to explore these emotional connections. Journaling or speaking with a therapist can be valuable tools for processing and releasing emotional pain.

Mindfulness in Complementary Therapies
Mindfulness can enhance the effectiveness of complementary therapies often used to manage chronic pain. When combined, these therapies can provide holistic relief. Here are some examples:

1. Yoga: The practice of yoga combines physical postures, breathing exercises, and meditation. When approached mindfully, it can improve flexibility, reduce muscle tension, and alleviate pain.

2. Acupuncture: Acupuncture, a traditional Chinese therapy, involves the insertion of thin needles into specific points on the body. Mindfulness meditation before and during acupuncture sessions can enhance the pain-relieving effects.

3. Massage Therapy: Mindfulness can make massage therapy more effective by helping you connect with your body and sensations. Communicate with your massage therapist about your pain and preferences.

4. Chiropractic Care: Chiropractic adjustments aim to restore proper alignment in the body. Mindfulness can complement this therapy by promoting relaxation and self-awareness, which can aid in pain reduction.

Incorporating mindfulness into these complementary therapies can amplify their benefits, offering you a multifaceted approach to managing chronic pain. Remember that the key to successful pain management through mindfulness is consistency. Over time, you'll develop a greater sense of control over your pain and experience improved overall well-being.

3.3 Mindful Living for Mental Health

Our mental health is connected to our physical well-being..
Yet, for far too long, we've treated these two aspects of our
existence as separate entities, failing to recognize the
profound interplay between mind and body. This
subchapter is dedicated to unraveling the mysteries of this
connection and exploring how mindfulness can serve as a
powerful tool for nurturing mental health, cultivating
resilience, and navigating the turbulent waters of trauma.

Mindfulness for Anxiety and Depression

Anxiety and depression are silent storms that can wreak
havoc on our mental well-being. They creep into our
minds, casting doubts, fears, and an overwhelming sense of
sadness. Yet, the practice of mindfulness serves as a
lighthouse, guiding us through the darkest of mental seas.

Mindfulness allows us to observe our thoughts and
emotions without judgment. It's about being fully present in
the moment, acknowledging whatever arises within us.
When anxiety tightens its grip, mindfulness encourages us
to breathe and acknowledge the anxiety, but not to be
consumed by it.

1: Observing Anxiety and Depression

The first step in using mindfulness for anxiety and
depression is awareness. When you feel the grip of anxiety
or the weight of depression, take a moment to pause. Sit
down, close your eyes, and breathe deeply. Allow yourself
to become fully aware of the sensations in your body.

Notice the tension in your muscles, the racing of your heart, or the heaviness in your chest.

2: Embracing Acceptance

The next step is acceptance. Accept that anxiety and depression are natural parts of the human experience. They do not define you, nor do they control your destiny. Instead of fighting these emotions, embrace them with kindness. Treat yourself as you would a dear friend in distress.

3: Mindful Release

Now, practice letting go. As you breathe deeply and accept your emotions, visualize them as passing clouds in the vast sky of your consciousness. Watch them drift away, knowing they will return from time to time, but that you possess the power to let them go again and again.

Cultivating Resilience through Mindful Living
Resilience is the art of bouncing back, not despite adversity, but because of it. Mindful living equips us with the tools to develop this crucial skill. Resilience is not about avoiding challenges; it's about learning how to face them with grace and courage.

Resilience starts with a mindset shift. Rather than viewing challenges as insurmountable obstacles, see them as opportunities for growth. When life throws you a curveball, pause and ask yourself, "What can I learn from this experience?" This shift in perspective can transform adversity into a stepping stone on your path to personal growth.

Resilience is not about toughening up; it's about being gentle with yourself. Practice self-compassion through mindful self-care. When you face setbacks or disappointments, treat yourself as you would a beloved friend. Offer yourself words of kindness and encouragement.

Daily mindfulness practices strengthen your mental resilience. Begin your day with a few moments of meditation or deep breathing. Throughout the day, pause to check in with yourself. Are you feeling stressed? Overwhelmed? Take a moment to ground yourself through mindful awareness.

Mindful Strategies for Dealing with Trauma
Trauma leaves deep imprints on our minds and bodies. It's like a wound that, if left unattended, can fester and affect every aspect of our lives. Mindfulness offers a gentle path toward healing from trauma.

1: Mindful Healing Space

Create a safe and healing space for yourself. This can be a physical place where you feel secure or a mental refuge you visit in times of distress. When you feel overwhelmed by traumatic memories or emotions, retreat to this space. Take

deep breaths and remind yourself that you are safe in this
moment.

2: Mindful Journaling

Journaling is a powerful tool for processing trauma.
Through mindful journaling, you can express your thoughts
and emotions without judgment. Take time each day to
write about your experiences, fears, and hopes. Allow your
journal to be a witness to your healing journey.

3: Mindful Support

You don't have to navigate the path of healing alone. Seek
support from a therapist or support group experienced in
trauma recovery. Mindful living includes recognizing when
it's time to reach out for help and accepting that it's a sign
of strength, not weakness.

The mind-body connection is a potent force in disease
prevention. By embracing mindfulness, we can confront
anxiety, depression, and trauma with courage and
resilience. Through mindfulness, we learn to observe our
emotions, cultivate resilience, and heal from past traumas.
Remember that you hold the power to transform your
mental landscape through the simple yet profound practice
of mindful living. Your journey towards greater mental
health and well-being starts with a single mindful breath.

Chapter 4: Mindful Nutrition and Disease Resilience

4.1 Mindful Eating Principles

In a world filled with fast food joints, tempting treats, and endless distractions, eating has become more of a rushed routine than a mindful act. We often consume our meals on autopilot, unaware of the intricate dance between our bodies and the food on our plates. But what if I told you that by rekindling the ancient art of mindful eating, you could pave the way for resilience against diseases and a harmonious relationship with food? Welcome to the realm of mindful nutrition, where every bite becomes an opportunity for wellness.

Mindful Awareness of Eating Habits

Let's start with the first and perhaps the most foundational principle of mindful eating: becoming aware of your eating habits. You see, our lives are often a whirlwind of activity, and it's easy to fall into the trap of mindless eating. We eat on autopilot, shoveling food into our mouths without really paying attention.

Mindful eating begins with mindfulness itself – being present in the moment, fully aware of your actions, sensations, and surroundings. When you sit down to eat, take a moment to pause and simply observe. Notice the colors, textures, and aromas of your food. Pay attention to the physical sensations in your body, like hunger and satiety cues.

Here's a practical step: Before you take that first bite, close your eyes for a moment and take a few deep breaths. This simple act can center you in the present moment, preparing you to eat with full awareness.

Mindful eating is a bit like pressing the pause button on your day. It allows you to break free from the hustle and bustle, to savor each bite, and to connect with the experience of nourishing your body. It's about putting away distractions – the TV, the phone, the endless stream of thoughts – and devoting your attention to your plate.

Mindful Portion Control and Food Choices
Now that you're fully present at your meal, let's delve into the next principle: mindful portion control and food choices. This isn't about restriction or rigid dieting; it's about making choices that align with your health and well-being while still enjoying the pleasures of eating.

Imagine your plate as a canvas, and each item of food as a color on that canvas. Mindful eating encourages you to paint your plate with a variety of colors – a medley of fruits, vegetables, whole grains, lean proteins, and healthy fats. By doing so, you ensure that you're getting a wide range of nutrients that support your body's resilience against diseases.

Practically speaking, this means filling half your plate with vegetables and fruits. The vibrant colors of these foods signal the presence of antioxidants, vitamins, and minerals that boost your immune system and protect against chronic illnesses. The remaining half of your plate can be shared between lean proteins and whole grains. Think of it as creating a balanced symphony of flavors and textures.

As for portion control, it's about tuning in to your body's hunger and fullness cues. Start with a smaller portion than you think you need, and savor each bite slowly. It takes about 20 minutes for your brain to register that you're full, so eating mindfully can help prevent overeating. If you're still hungry after finishing your initial portion, take a few minutes before deciding if you want seconds. This pause gives your body time to communicate its needs.

Mindful Eating for Weight Management
One of the beautiful outcomes of mindful eating is its impact on weight management. When you eat mindfully, you're less likely to consume excess calories, emotional eating becomes less of a crutch, and you're better equipped to respond to your body's true hunger cues.

But here's the thing: mindful eating is not a crash diet or a quick fix. It's a sustainable approach to nourishing your body. When you consistently practice mindful eating, you develop a deeper connection with your body's signals. You begin to discern whether you're eating out of genuine hunger or for emotional reasons.

Let's put this into action. The next time you find yourself reaching for a snack, pause for a moment and ask yourself, "Am I really hungry, or am I eating to fill an emotional void?" If it's emotional, try to identify the emotion – is it stress, boredom, sadness? Then, consider alternative ways to address that emotion that don't involve food. Maybe it's a short walk, a phone call to a friend, or a few minutes of deep breathing.

Another practical step is to keep a food journal. Not as a means of calorie counting, but as a way to record what you eat, when you eat, and how you feel before and after. This simple practice can help you uncover patterns in your eating habits and identify areas for improvement.

The beauty of mindful eating for weight management is that it allows you to enjoy your favorite foods without guilt. It's about savoring every bite, experiencing the pleasure of food, and making choices that honor your body's needs.

Incorporating these mindful eating principles into your daily life is a powerful step toward disease resilience and overall well-being. By embracing it at the table, you're not only nourishing your body but also cultivating a deeper connection with yourself and the food you consume. Your path to a resilient, disease-fighting diet starts with awareness, balance, and mindfulness.

4.2 Mindful Nutrition for Specific Health Goals

In our journey toward better health through mindful living, few aspects hold as much significance as nutrition. What we put into our bodies isn't just fuel; it's the foundation upon which our well-being is built. In this subchapter, we'll explore the transformative power of mindful nutrition for specific health goals—particularly, how you can use it to fortify your heart, prevent or manage diabetes, and nurture a healthier digestive system.

Mindful Eating for Heart Health

Your heart, that remarkable organ tirelessly pumping life through your veins, deserves your utmost care and attention. And the food you choose plays a pivotal role in its well-being. Mindful eating for heart health isn't just about what you should avoid; it's about embracing a lifestyle that truly nourishes your most vital organ.

1: Heart-Healthy Food Choices

Heart-healthy eating starts with wise choices. Opt for foods rich in omega-3 fatty acids, like salmon, flaxseeds, and walnuts. These little powerhouses can help lower your cholesterol levels and reduce inflammation within your arteries.

Additionally, consider introducing more leafy greens into your diet. Spinach, kale, and Swiss chard provide a wealth of vitamins, minerals, and antioxidants that promote heart health. And don't forget the power of fiber. Whole grains, such as oats, quinoa, and brown rice, help lower cholesterol and maintain stable blood sugar levels.

2: Portion Control and Mindful Eating Habits

Mindful eating isn't just about what you eat but also about how you eat. Slow down and savor your meals. Enjoy each bite, appreciating the flavors, textures, and aromas. This practice not only enhances your dining experience but also helps prevent overeating.

Furthermore, portion control is essential. Avoid those all-you-can-eat buffet mentality. Serve yourself smaller portions, and, if you're still hungry, you can always have more. This simple practice can go a long way in maintaining a healthy weight and preventing heart-related issues.

3: Limiting Sodium and Processed Foods

Excessive sodium intake is a major contributor to high blood pressure, a significant risk factor for heart disease. Be vigilant about reading food labels and reducing your sodium intake. Opt for fresh, whole foods over highly processed alternatives.

Consider swapping out that salt shaker for herbs and spices to flavor your meals. Not only will you enhance the taste of your food, but you'll also lower your sodium consumption. Your heart will thank you for it.

Mindful Nutrition for Diabetes Prevention and Management

Diabetes is a prevalent and often preventable condition that affects millions worldwide. The good news is that mindful nutrition can be a potent tool for both preventing the onset of diabetes and effectively managing it if you've already been diagnosed.

1: Embracing Whole, Unprocessed Foods

Whole foods are a diabetes warrior's best friend. These unprocessed, natural gems help stabilize blood sugar levels and reduce the risk of developing type 2 diabetes. Incorporate more fruits, vegetables, whole grains, lean proteins, and legumes into your diet.

Fiber-rich foods, like beans, lentils, and oats, are particularly beneficial for managing blood sugar levels. They slow down digestion, preventing rapid spikes in blood glucose. Additionally, fiber keeps you feeling fuller for longer, aiding in weight management—a critical aspect of diabetes prevention and control.

2: Balanced Carbohydrate Consumption

Carbohydrates play a central role in diabetes management. It's not about cutting carbs altogether but rather choosing them wisely. Opt for complex carbohydrates with a low glycemic index, like sweet potatoes, quinoa, and whole wheat bread.

Mindful carb portioning is vital. Pay attention to your body's response to different foods. Monitor how specific carbohydrates affect your blood sugar levels, and adjust your choices accordingly. Remember, there's no one-size-fits-all approach to diabetes nutrition.

3: Monitoring Blood Sugar and Staying Hydrated

Regularly monitoring your blood sugar levels is paramount for diabetes management. It allows you to make informed decisions about your diet and medication. Additionally, stay well-hydrated, as dehydration can affect blood sugar control.

Remember that beverages can impact your blood sugar, too. Opt for water, herbal tea, or unsweetened beverages whenever possible. Sugary drinks can lead to rapid blood sugar spikes and should be consumed sparingly or avoided entirely.

Mindful Eating for Digestive Health
A healthy digestive system is the cornerstone of overall well-being. It ensures the efficient absorption of nutrients and the elimination of waste. Mindful nutrition can significantly influence the health of your digestive tract.

1: Embracing Gut-Friendly Foods

Your gut is home to a diverse community of microorganisms, collectively known as the microbiota. A diet rich in fiber, prebiotics (found in foods like garlic, onions, and bananas), and probiotics (found in fermented foods like yogurt and kefir) supports a thriving microbiota.

These beneficial bacteria not only aid digestion but also contribute to a robust immune system and even impact your mood and mental health. Incorporating these foods into your diet can lead to a happier, healthier gut.

2: Hydration and Fiber for Regularity

Proper hydration is essential for maintaining regular bowel movements. Water softens stool, making it easier to pass. Alongside hydration, dietary fiber is key for digestive regularity.

Increase your fiber intake through whole grains, fruits, and vegetables. Fiber adds bulk to your stool, preventing constipation and promoting healthy bowel movements. Be sure to gradually introduce more fiber into your diet to avoid digestive discomfort.

3: Mindful Eating Practices for Digestion

Mindful eating extends to your digestive processes. Chewing your food thoroughly aids digestion, allowing enzymes in your saliva to begin breaking down carbohydrates. Eating slowly and savoring your meals not only enhances the dining experience but also aids digestion.

Avoid overeating, as it can strain your digestive system. Eating until you're comfortably satisfied, not uncomfortably full, is a mindful practice that supports your digestive health.

Mindful nutrition is a powerful tool for promoting disease resilience and overall well-being. By making thoughtful choices, embracing whole, unprocessed foods, and adopting mindful eating habits, you can fortify your heart, prevent or manage diabetes, and nurture a healthier digestive system. These practical steps can lead to a happier, healthier you, ready to tackle life's challenges with vitality and resilience.

4.3 Mindful Meal Planning and Preparation

In the quest for disease resilience and overall health, one of the most potent tools at our disposal is mindful nutrition. What we eat plays a pivotal role in shaping our well-being, and by embracing the principles of mindful meal planning and preparation, we can harness the transformative power of food. In this subchapter, we will explore the art of creating balanced and nutritious meals mindfully, navigating the aisles with mindful grocery shopping, and employing mindful cooking techniques for optimal health.

Creating Balanced and Nutritious Meals Mindfully
The cornerstone of a healthy diet lies in the meals we put
on our plates. Creating balanced and nutritious meals
requires mindfulness at every stage, from planning to
plating. Let's delve into the practical steps you can take to
ensure that each meal is a nourishing experience:

1. Mindful Meal Planning:

   - Begin by setting aside dedicated time for meal planning.
This act alone can make a significant difference in your
dietary choices.

   - Consider your nutritional needs and goals. Are you
looking to boost your immune system, manage your
weight, or enhance your energy levels? Tailor your meals
accordingly.

   - Prioritize variety. Incorporate a rainbow of fruits and
vegetables, whole grains, lean proteins, and healthy fats
into your weekly menu.

   - Create a meal plan for the week ahead, taking into
account your schedule and cooking preferences. Having a
plan reduces the temptation to resort to less healthy options
on busy days.

   - Experiment with new recipes and cuisines to keep your
meals exciting and enjoyable.

2. Mindful Portion Control:

- Pay attention to portion sizes. Mindful eating includes being aware of when you're satisfied and stopping before you're overly full.

- Utilize smaller plates and utensils to naturally reduce portion sizes.

- Listen to your body's hunger and fullness cues. Eat slowly and savor each bite, allowing your brain to register when you're no longer hungry.

- Consider using mindful eating apps or journals to track your eating habits and emotional triggers.

3. Mindful Ingredient Selection:

- Read food labels carefully. Look for hidden sugars, excessive sodium, and unhealthy trans fats.

- Choose whole, unprocessed foods whenever possible. These are often richer in essential nutrients and lower in additives.

- Be discerning about added sauces, dressings, and condiments, as they can contribute hidden calories and unhealthy fats.

Mindful Grocery Shopping and Food Labeling
Your journey toward mindful nutrition starts long before you reach your kitchen. It begins in the aisles of your local

grocery store, where you have the opportunity to make choices that support your health and resilience.

1. Plan Your Shopping Trip:

   - Make a shopping list based on your meal plan. Having a list helps you stay focused and avoid impulse purchases.

   - Shop after a meal or snack to reduce the temptation to buy unhealthy foods when you're hungry.

   - Choose a time when the store is less crowded to minimize stress and distractions.

2. Navigating the Aisles Mindfully:

   - Start your shopping journey in the produce section. Load up on fresh fruits and vegetables, aiming for a colorful variety.

   - Explore the perimeter of the store, where you'll find fresh foods like dairy, meats, and bakery items. This is often where the healthiest options are located.

   - Practice label reading. Check for ingredients, nutrition facts, and any potential allergens or additives.

   - When choosing packaged foods, opt for those with shorter ingredient lists and recognizable ingredients.

   - Don't forget to visit the bulk section for whole grains, nuts, and seeds, which are often more cost-effective and less processed.

3. Mindful Shopping Habits:

  - Stick to your shopping list as closely as possible to avoid unnecessary purchases.

  - Be mindful of sales and discounts. Sometimes, buying in bulk or choosing store brands can be more cost-effective.

  - Consider shopping online or using grocery delivery services if they are available in your area. Online shopping can help you avoid impulsive purchases and stick to your list.

Mindful Cooking Techniques for Optimal Health
With a well-planned meal and a cart full of nutritious ingredients, it's time to transform these raw materials into delicious, healthful dishes. Mindful cooking is about savoring the process as much as the end result.

  1. Preparation Mindfulness:

  - Begin by organizing your ingredients and tools before you start cooking. This minimizes stress during the cooking process.

  - Practice mise en place, a French culinary term that means "everything in its place." Having all your ingredients measured, chopped, and ready to go before you start cooking makes the process smoother and more enjoyable.

  - Engage your senses as you prepare your ingredients. Take a moment to appreciate the aroma of herbs, the

texture of vegetables, and the vibrant colors of your
ingredients.

2. Mindful Cooking Methods:

   - Opt for cooking methods that retain the nutritional value
of your ingredients, such as steaming, roasting, or sautéing
in healthy fats like olive oil.

   - Minimize the use of excessive oils, salt, and sugar.
Experiment with herbs and spices to add flavor and depth
to your dishes.

   - Pay attention to cooking times to prevent overcooking,
which can result in nutrient loss and less appealing textures.

   - Use cooking techniques that preserve the integrity of
your ingredients. For example, stir-frying can maintain the
vibrant colors and crispness of vegetables.

3. Savoring the Finished Dish:

   - Once your meal is ready, serve it on a clean, attractive
plate. Presentation can enhance your appreciation of the
meal.

   - Eat mindfully, savoring each bite. Put away distractions
like phones or screens to fully engage with your food.

- Take breaks between bites to assess your hunger and fullness cues. This practice can help prevent overeating and promote a healthier relationship with food.

By approaching meal planning, grocery shopping, and cooking with mindfulness, you not only nourish your body but also cultivate a deeper connection to the food you consume. These practices can lead to improved disease resilience, enhanced well-being, and a more profound sense of satisfaction with your diet. Remember, it's not just about what you eat but how you eat it that makes a difference in your health journey.

Chapter 5: Fasting and Mental Health

5.1 Fasting and Mood Regulation

In the quest for a healthier, more vibrant life, we often focus on the physical aspects—weight loss, disease prevention, and longevity. However, we sometimes forget that our mental well-being is just as crucial, if not more so. Our emotional stability and mood play an integral role in our overall health and happiness. Surprisingly, fasting can be a powerful tool for enhancing our mood and emotional resilience.

Fasting's Impact on Mood and Emotional Stability

When we talk about fasting and mood regulation, it's essential to understand that our bodies and minds are intricately linked. What you put into your body affects how you feel emotionally. Fasting, in particular, can be a game-changer.

Fasting is like hitting the reset button for your brain. It initiates a cascade of biological processes that help your brain function more efficiently. When you abstain from food for a certain period, your body begins to tap into its energy reserves, primarily stored as glycogen and fat. As this process unfolds, something fascinating happens: your brain starts producing more neurotrophic factors like brain-derived neurotrophic factor (BDNF). This is your brain's natural fertilizer for growth and repair.

BDNF is responsible for enhancing synaptic connections, boosting mood, and reducing the risk of depression. So, during fasting, your brain is essentially upgrading its own software, leading to improved emotional resilience.

But it's not just about BDNF. Fasting also triggers the release of endorphins, your body's natural mood elevators. You've probably heard of the "runner's high," right? Well, fasting can induce a similar feeling of euphoria. As your body adapts to the fasting state, it becomes more efficient at releasing these feel-good chemicals.

So, here's the practical takeaway: By incorporating fasting into your routine, you're not only giving your body a physical detox but also providing your brain with the tools it needs to boost your mood and enhance emotional stability.

Strategies for Fasting-Related Mood Management
Now that you know fasting's potential to brighten your emotional landscape, let's discuss some practical strategies for making the most of it:

1. Start Slowly: If you're new to fasting, don't dive headfirst into an extended fast. Begin with intermittent fasting, where you restrict your eating window to a specific time frame (e.g., 16/8 fasting). Gradually extend the fasting duration as you become more comfortable.

2. Stay Hydrated: Dehydration can affect your mood negatively. Make sure you're drinking plenty of water, herbal teas, or black coffee during your fasting periods to stay hydrated.

3. Monitor Your Energy: Pay attention to your body's signals. If you're feeling weak, dizzy, or excessively irritable during a fast, it might be a sign that it's time to eat. Fasting should enhance your mood, not leave you feeling miserable.

4. Combine Fasting with Nutrient-Dense Foods: When you do eat, opt for nutrient-rich, whole foods. Avoid highly processed and sugary foods that can cause mood swings.

5. Incorporate Mindfulness: Mindfulness isn't just for meditation; it can be applied to eating as well. When you do break your fast, do it mindfully. Savor each bite, and be fully present during your meal. This can help you appreciate the nourishment and enhance your mood.

Mindfulness Techniques During Fasting for Mental Well-being

Let's talk about the secret sauce to supercharge your fasting journey: mindfulness. Combining mindfulness practices with fasting can be a game-changer for your mental well-being.

Mindful Breathing: One of the simplest and most effective mindfulness techniques is mindful breathing. During your fasting hours, take a few moments to focus on your breath. Inhale deeply, counting to four, hold for four counts, and exhale for four counts. This simple exercise can help calm your mind and reduce stress, making fasting more manageable.

Body Scan Meditation: Another powerful tool is the body scan meditation. Start at the top of your head and slowly move your attention down through your body, noticing any tension or discomfort. This practice can help you become more in tune with your body's needs during fasting and alleviate emotional stress.

Positive Affirmations: During fasting, negative thoughts or doubts might creep in. Combat them with positive affirmations. Remind yourself why you're fasting and the benefits you're reaping. This mental shift can have a profound impact on your mood and motivation.

Incorporating these mindfulness techniques into your fasting routine can elevate your emotional well-being and make the process more enjoyable. Remember, fasting is not just about physical transformation; it's a holistic journey that can enhance your mental health, too.

Fasting and mood regulation are two sides of the same coin. When done mindfully and with intention, fasting can become a powerful tool to boost your emotional stability and overall mental well-being. So, embrace this journey, stay mindful, and watch as your mood soars to new heights.

5.2 Fasting and Cognitive Health

In the quest for optimal health and well-being, we sometimes overlooking the incredible influence that fasting can have on our mental health and cognitive function. Our brain is a remarkable organ, and its health profoundly impacts every aspect of our lives, from decision-making and problem-solving to emotional regulation and creativity. In this subchapter, we will delve into the intriguing connection between fasting and cognitive health, exploring how fasting can enhance brain function and protect it from the rigors of modern life.

Fasting's Influence on Brain Function and Cognitive Enhancement

Our brains are dynamic and adaptive, constantly changing in response to our environment and lifestyle choices. Fasting, it turns out, can serve as a powerful catalyst for cognitive enhancement. Let's uncover how:

1. Enhancing Brain-Derived Neurotrophic Factor (BDNF): Fasting triggers the release of a remarkable protein known as Brain-Derived Neurotrophic Factor, or BDNF. This protein acts like fertilizer for our brain cells, promoting the growth of new neurons and strengthening existing connections. As BDNF levels rise during fasting, our brain's plasticity increases, allowing us to learn more efficiently and adapt to new challenges.

2. Improved Brain Energy: When we fast, our bodies switch from using glucose as a primary energy source to burning fat. This metabolic shift benefits our brain in

multiple ways. Ketones, produced during fasting, provide a highly efficient fuel for brain cells. This heightened energy supply improves cognitive performance, enhancing focus, and mental clarity.

3. Reducing Inflammation: Chronic inflammation in the body can have devastating effects on cognitive function. Fasting helps reduce inflammation, not only in the body but also in the brain. By lowering inflammatory markers, fasting contributes to a calmer, more resilient mind, less susceptible to stress-induced cognitive decline.

Mindful Living Practices for Improved Cognitive Health

While fasting itself is a potent tool for cognitive enhancement, combining it with mindful living practices can supercharge the benefits. Here's how to harness the power of both:

1. Mindful Eating During Fasting: When it's time to break your fast, do so mindfully. Savor each bite, paying full attention to the flavors, textures, and sensations. This practice not only enhances your appreciation of food but also supports cognitive health. Mindful eating has been shown to improve memory and reduce overeating, ensuring that you provide your brain with the nourishment it needs.

2. Daily Meditation: Regular meditation is a cornerstone of mindful living and has profound effects on cognitive health. Meditation reduces stress, calms the mind, and enhances focus. Consider incorporating a brief meditation

session into your daily routine, especially during fasting periods. This practice will fortify your cognitive resilience and sharpen your mental faculties.

3. Stay Hydrated: Dehydration can impair cognitive function, leading to decreased focus and alertness. During fasting, it's essential to stay adequately hydrated. Water is the elixir of life for your brain, ensuring that it operates at its peak. Add a slice of lemon or cucumber for a refreshing twist, but avoid sugary beverages that can disrupt mental clarity.

The Role of Fasting in Neuroprotection
Beyond cognitive enhancement, fasting offers a unique form of neuroprotection, shielding our brains from the ravages of time and external stressors. Here's how fasting becomes a guardian of your most vital organ:

1. Autophagy and Cellular Clean-Up: Fasting promotes a process called autophagy, which can be thought of as a cellular cleaning crew. During autophagy, cells identify and remove damaged components, including those in the brain. This process helps prevent the accumulation of toxic proteins associated with neurodegenerative diseases, such as Alzheimer's and Parkinson's.

2. Enhanced Brain Resilience: Fasting induces a mild stress response in the brain, similar to the beneficial stress of exercise. This eustress, or positive stress, strengthens neuronal pathways and enhances the brain's ability to adapt and cope with future challenges. In essence, fasting

toughens up your brain, making it more resilient in the face of adversity.

3. Protection Against Cognitive Decline: Neurological conditions like Alzheimer's disease often involve the accumulation of beta-amyloid plaques. Fasting may help reduce the buildup of these plaques, potentially delaying the onset of cognitive decline and preserving your cognitive faculties as you age.

Incorporating fasting into your life, along with mindful living practices, can be a game-changer for your cognitive health. It's a practical and actionable step toward unlocking your brain's full potential while safeguarding it against the challenges of our fast-paced world. Embrace these practices with intention and dedication, and you'll find yourself on a path to enhanced cognitive function, mental clarity, and a sharper mind for life.

5.3 Combining Mindful Living and Fasting for Psychological Resilience

In the quest for better mental health, we often overlook the profound connection between what we eat and how we feel. Fasting, when combined with mindful living, can become a powerful ally in building psychological resilience, fostering emotional stability, and helping us navigate life's challenges with grace and poise. In this subchapter, we'll explore how to harness the combined power of mindful living and fasting to strengthen your mental fortitude, build a supportive community, and effectively manage cravings and emotional eating.

Synergizing mindfulness and fasting for emotional resilience

Let's begin by understanding the synergy between mindfulness and fasting when it comes to emotional resilience. Mindfulness is the art of being fully present in the moment, accepting it without judgment. It equips us with the mental tools to manage stress, anxiety, and negative emotions, which are all too common in today's fast-paced world.

Fasting, on the other hand, teaches us discipline and self-control. It asks us to confront our cravings, our relationship with food, and our emotional triggers head-on. But here's the magic: when you pair mindfulness with fasting, you create a dynamic duo that empowers you to observe your cravings without judgment. You become an observer of your emotions, not a victim of them.

When fasting, those hunger pangs and cravings for your favorite snacks may surface, especially during the initial stages. But by incorporating mindfulness, you can watch these sensations and thoughts arise without reacting impulsively. This teaches you to pause, breathe, and explore the root cause of your cravings. Are you hungry for food, or is it an emotional hunger, perhaps a response to stress or boredom? By observing without judgment, you gain insight into your relationship with food and emotions.

Building a supportive mindful community during fasting

Fasting can be a solitary journey, but it doesn't have to be. Humans are social beings, and sharing our experiences can be profoundly therapeutic. Building a mindful community during your fasting journey can provide the emotional support, encouragement, and camaraderie needed to stay the course.

Reach out to friends, family members, or join online groups of individuals who share your interest in fasting and mindfulness. Share your experiences, challenges, and triumphs. By doing so, you create a network of support that understands your journey intimately. You'll find strength in knowing that you're not alone in your quest for emotional resilience through fasting and mindfulness.

Mindfulness for managing cravings and emotional eating

Cravings are powerful, often leading us to make impulsive and unhealthy food choices. Whether it's stress, sadness, or even joy, emotions can trigger these cravings. But the combination of mindfulness and fasting arms you with potent tools to manage them effectively.

Mindful eating helps you savor the flavors, textures, and aromas of your food, bringing your focus to the present moment. When you practice mindful eating during your eating windows in a fasting regimen, you not only enhance your enjoyment of food but also gain better control over emotional eating.

Before you eat, take a moment to pause and breathe. Observe the thoughts and emotions that arise. Are you eating because you're genuinely hungry, or is it a reaction to stress or another emotion? Mindful eating allows you to distinguish between physical hunger and emotional hunger, making it easier to make conscious, nourishing choices.

By being fully present during your meals, you reduce the chances of overeating or making unhealthy food choices driven by emotions. This practice not only helps you maintain a healthy weight but also cultivates emotional intelligence, strengthening your ability to manage emotional triggers in daily life.

Combining mindful living and fasting creates a potent recipe for psychological resilience. The synergy between these two practices allows you to observe your cravings without judgment, build a supportive community, and use mindfulness to manage emotional eating. Every mindful choice you make brings you one step closer to a resilient, emotionally balanced life.

Chapter 6: Mindful Movement for Physical Wellness

6.1 Mindful Exercise Approaches

In our modern, fast-paced lives, exercise is often seen as a means to an end—an activity that serves the purpose of staying fit or losing weight. We hit the gym, go for a run, or engage in various forms of physical activity with a clear objective in mind. While there's nothing wrong with setting fitness goals, we often overlook a fundamental aspect of exercise—mindful movement.

Mindful Awareness in Physical Activity

Let's begin our journey into mindful exercise by exploring the first key point: mindful awareness in physical activity.

Mindful awareness is the practice of being fully present in the moment, paying attention to your thoughts, feelings, and bodily sensations without judgment. In the context of exercise, it means immersing yourself in the experience of movement, rather than treating it as a chore or a means to an end.

To start, find an activity you genuinely enjoy. It could be anything from yoga and dancing to hiking and cycling. The key is to choose something that resonates with you, something that makes you look forward to moving your body.

When you engage in this activity, be fully present. Pay attention to the rhythm of your breath, the sensation of your muscles contracting and relaxing, and the way your body moves through space. Notice the sights, sounds, and smells around you. Allow yourself to become absorbed in the experience.

As you develop this mindful awareness during exercise, you'll likely notice several benefits. First, you'll find that time flies by as you become fully engaged in the activity. This makes exercise more enjoyable, which means you're more likely to stick with it in the long run.

Second, you'll gain a deeper understanding of your body. You'll start to notice subtle cues, like when your posture is off or when you're tensing up unnecessarily. This awareness can help prevent injuries and improve your overall form.

Mindful Techniques for Stress Reduction During Exercise
The second key point of mindful exercise involves using movement as a tool for stress reduction.

We all experience stress in our lives, and exercise can be a powerful antidote. However, to make the most of this stress-relieving potential, we need to approach exercise mindfully.

Start by setting an intention before your workout. Instead of focusing solely on physical outcomes like burning calories or building muscle, consider what you want to achieve mentally and emotionally. Is it stress relief, mental clarity, or a sense of calm? By setting an intention, you're creating a purpose for your exercise that goes beyond the physical.

As you move, pay attention to how your body responds to stress. Notice if you tend to clench your jaw, furrow your brow, or hold tension in your shoulders. When you catch yourself doing this, consciously release the tension. Soften your facial muscles, relax your shoulders, and take a few deep breaths.

Another effective technique for stress reduction during exercise is syncing your breath with your movements. For example, in yoga, each pose is often paired with a specific breath pattern. This synchronization not only enhances the mind-body connection but also regulates your nervous system, promoting relaxation.

Lastly, practice gratitude during your workout. As you move, express appreciation for your body's abilities and the opportunity to be active. Gratitude has a profound impact on our mental well-being, and incorporating it into exercise can turn a routine workout into a joyful experience.

Integrating Mindfulness into Various Exercise Routines

Now that we've covered the importance of mindful awareness and stress reduction during exercise, let's explore how you can integrate mindfulness into different types of workouts.

1. Yoga: Yoga is an excellent example of a mindful exercise. Each pose requires focused attention on

alignment, balance, and breath. Whether you're practicing
Hatha, Vinyasa, or any other style, approach it with the
intention of mindfulness. Notice how each pose feels in
your body, and let go of distractions.

2. Running or Walking: These activities offer a perfect
opportunity for mindfulness. Pay attention to the sensation
of your feet hitting the ground, the rhythm of your breath,
and the scenery around you. Consider leaving your
headphones at home occasionally to fully immerse yourself
in the experience.

3. Strength Training: Even in the world of weights and
resistance, mindfulness has a place. Focus on the quality of
your movements rather than the quantity of repetitions.
Feel the muscles engaging and releasing with each lift.
Concentrate on your breath to maintain form and prevent
unnecessary strain.

4. Dance: Whether you're a professional dancer or just
dancing in your living room, embrace the moment. Let the
music guide your movements, and express yourself fully.
Dancing mindfully is a fantastic way to release pent-up
emotions and boost your mood.

5. Hiking or Nature Walks: If you're fortunate enough to
have access to nature, take advantage of it. Hiking or
simply walking in natural surroundings can be incredibly
grounding. Use all your senses to connect with the
environment, from the rustling leaves to the scent of the
forest.

Incorporating mindfulness into your exercise routine doesn't require any special equipment or a particular setting. It's a mindset you can carry with you wherever you move your body. Over time, you'll find that mindful exercise not only enhances physical well-being but also fosters mental clarity and emotional balance. Embrace the process, savor the moments of presence, and let your exercise routine become a sacred space for self-discovery and well-being.

6.2 Mindful Movement and Pain Management

Pain is an unwelcome companion that can disrupt our lives in various ways. Whether it's chronic pain from an old injury or the occasional twinge from strenuous activity, pain can be debilitating. But here's the good news: mindful movement can be a powerful ally in managing and even alleviating pain. In this subchapter, we'll explore practical, actionable steps to harness the therapeutic potential of mindful movement for pain relief.

Mindful Practices for Pain Relief During Movement

Pain often triggers a natural response to avoid movement. It's as if our bodies are saying, "Stop! Don't move, it hurts!" However, this avoidance can lead to stiffness and further discomfort. The key is to approach movement mindfully, acknowledging pain while gradually working to alleviate it.

1. Breath as Your Guide: Start by taking a few moments to focus on your breath. As you inhale and exhale, visualize the breath flowing to the areas of pain. With each breath, imagine releasing tension and discomfort. This simple act of mindfulness can help relax your body and prepare it for movement.

2. Gentle Range of Motion: Begin with gentle, slow movements within your pain-free range of motion. For example, if you have knee pain, gently bend and extend your knee without pushing into the pain. As you move, focus your attention on the sensations and any changes in discomfort.

3. Progressive Muscle Relaxation: As you continue to move, pay attention to the muscles around the painful area. Imagine them relaxing with each movement. This mental focus on relaxation can help reduce muscle tension that often accompanies pain.

4. Mindful Observation: Observe the pain without judgment. Instead of labeling it as "bad" or "intolerable," approach it with curiosity. What does it feel like? Is it constant or does it change with movement? By mindfully observing your pain, you may gain insights into its nature.

5. Visualization: Use the power of visualization to guide your movements. Imagine your body healing as you move. Visualize a warm, soothing light enveloping the painful area, gradually reducing discomfort.

Mindful Postures and Stretches for Specific Ailments

Different types of pain require tailored approaches. Here are some mindful postures and stretches for specific common ailments:

1. Lower Back Pain:

   - Mindful Cat-Cow Stretch: Start on your hands and knees. Inhale as you arch your back (Cow), and exhale as you round it (Cat). Focus on the flow of breath and gentle spinal movement.

2. Neck and Shoulder Tension:

   - Mindful Neck Stretch: Gently tilt your head to one side, feeling a stretch along the neck and shoulder. Breathe deeply, and then switch to the other side.

3. Arthritis Pain:

   - Mindful Joint Circles: Rotate affected joints, such as wrists or ankles, in a circular motion. Imagine releasing stiffness and promoting lubrication within the joint.

4. Knee Pain:

   - Mindful Quadriceps Stretch: While standing, bend your knee and bring your heel toward your buttocks. Hold your ankle with your hand, feeling the stretch in the front of your thigh. Remember to breathe deeply and mindfully.

5. Headaches:

- Mindful Neck and Shoulder Release: Sit comfortably and gently tilt your head forward, feeling a stretch in the back of your neck. Hold the position while breathing deeply. This can alleviate tension headaches.

Mindful Body Awareness for Injury Prevention

Prevention is always better than cure, and mindful movement plays a crucial role in injury prevention. By developing body awareness and using proper alignment, you can reduce the risk of injuries during physical activities.

1. Start with a Body Scan: Before any physical activity, take a moment to scan your body. Pay attention to any areas of tension or discomfort. This self-awareness can help you identify potential problem areas.

2. Proper Alignment: Whether you're lifting weights, running, or doing yoga, pay close attention to your body's alignment. Maintain good posture and body mechanics to avoid unnecessary strain.

3. Mindful Warm-Up: Prioritize a mindful warm-up routine that includes dynamic stretches. This prepares your muscles and joints for more extensive movement, reducing the risk of injury.

4. Listen to Your Body: If you feel pain during an activity, don't push through it. Listen to your body's signals and modify or stop the movement if needed. It's crucial to distinguish between the discomfort of stretching and the pain of potential injury.

5. Balance and Coordination: Mindful movement also involves improving balance and coordination. Practices like tai chi and yoga can enhance these aspects, reducing the likelihood of trips, falls, and injuries.

Incorporating mindful movement into your daily routine can be transformative. Not only does it offer pain relief and injury prevention, but it also fosters a deeper connection between your mind and body. By approaching movement with mindfulness, you empower yourself to make informed choices that support your physical well-being.

6.3 Mindful Movement for Longevity and Vitality

Longevity and vitality are not just about living longer but living better—maintaining physical function, mental clarity, and emotional well-being as we age. In this subchapter, we delve into the profound connection between mindful movement and the art of graceful aging. It's not about chasing the fountain of youth; it's about embracing the present moment and moving with intention to nurture your body and soul.

How Mindful Movement Promotes Longevity

Longevity, the dream of living a healthy and fulfilling life well into our later years, is a goal many of us share. While genetics play a role, our lifestyle choices have an equally significant impact. Mindful movement, the deliberate practice of moving with awareness and intention, can be your secret weapon in this quest for a long and vibrant life.

As we age, our bodies naturally undergo changes. Muscle mass tends to decrease, joints may stiffen, and our overall flexibility can decline. However, mindful movement has the power to counteract these effects. It promotes longevity by preserving and enhancing the body's physical functions.

One key element of mindful movement is the cultivation of body awareness. When you move with mindfulness, you pay attention to how your body feels in each moment. You notice tension, discomfort, or areas of weakness. By identifying these areas, you can address them proactively, preventing issues from escalating into chronic conditions.

Mindful movement also encourages the development of a deep mind-body connection. Through this connection, you gain a heightened awareness of your body's limitations and capabilities. You learn to move in ways that respect your body's unique needs, reducing the risk of injury and strain.

Incorporating mindful movement into your daily routine can also help you maintain a healthy weight and prevent muscle loss. It engages your muscles and elevates your heart rate, contributing to improved cardiovascular health. As a result, you'll be better equipped to fend off diseases associated with aging, such as heart disease and diabetes.

Moreover, mindful movement supports brain health, promoting cognitive longevity. Studies have shown that regular physical activity, coupled with mindfulness, enhances cognitive function and memory. This means that not only will you feel younger, but you'll also think and remember more clearly as you age.

Enhancing Flexibility and Balance Through Mindfulness

Flexibility and balance are two pillars of physical wellness, especially as we grow older. They're not just about touching your toes or standing on one foot; they're about maintaining independence and preventing falls and injuries. Mindful movement offers a path to enhance both flexibility and balance, supporting your journey toward graceful aging.

When we speak of flexibility in mindful movement, we're not necessarily talking about becoming a contortionist. Instead, it's about improving your range of motion, which can make everyday tasks easier and more enjoyable. Mindfulness encourages you to explore your body's movement patterns gently and gradually, working to expand your flexibility over time.

One of the keys to achieving greater flexibility through mindful movement is the emphasis on relaxation. By learning to relax into your stretches and movements, you allow your muscles to release tension, making it easier to increase your range of motion. This approach minimizes the risk of injury and promotes a sense of ease in your body.

Balance, on the other hand, is a skill that can deteriorate with age if not actively maintained. Mindful movement practices, such as tai chi and yoga, are excellent tools for enhancing balance. These practices require a heightened awareness of your body's position in space, forcing you to engage and strengthen stabilizing muscles.

As you progress in your mindful movement journey, you'll likely notice improvements in your balance that extend beyond the mat or studio. You'll find it easier to maintain your equilibrium during everyday activities, reducing the risk of trips and falls.

Mindfulness also teaches you to be present in the moment, which is crucial for maintaining balance. When you're aware of your body's movements, you can adjust in real-time to prevent stumbles and accidents. This heightened awareness extends to your surroundings, making you more attuned to potential hazards.

Mindful Movement and the Connection to Graceful Aging

Graceful aging isn't just about looking good as you grow older; it's about feeling good and living a life of vitality. Mindful movement plays a pivotal role in achieving this graceful aging by helping you move with intention, awareness, and purpose.

One of the beautiful aspects of mindful movement is its adaptability. Regardless of your age or current physical condition, you can start a mindful movement practice today and reap its benefits immediately. The practices can be tailored to your individual needs and limitations, ensuring that you can engage in them at any stage of life.

As you age, mindful movement becomes a form of self-care that you can rely on to maintain your physical and mental well-being. It becomes a cherished routine that keeps you connected to your body and helps you navigate the inevitable changes that come with getting older.

Moreover, mindful movement fosters a sense of joy in physical activity. Unlike traditional exercise routines that may feel like a chore, mindful movement allows you to savor each movement, making it a pleasurable experience. This joy encourages consistency, which is key to reaping the long-term benefits of graceful aging.

The path to longevity and vitality can be paved with mindful movement. It promotes longevity by preserving and enhancing physical functions, enhances flexibility and balance through relaxation and awareness, and connects you to the art of graceful aging. By incorporating mindful movement into your life, you'll not only add years to your life but life to your years. It's a journey of self-discovery, self-care, and self-celebration that will empower you to age with grace and vitality.

Chapter 7: Fasting and Mindfulness for Longevity

7.1 Fasting and Cellular Aging

In the quest for longevity and the pursuit of a vibrant, healthy life, we often stumble upon age-old practices that promise to unlock the secrets of aging gracefully. One such practice, fasting, has gained significant attention in recent years for its potential to not only extend our lifespan but also enhance our overall well-being. As we delve into the fascinating realm of fasting and longevity, we'll explore its profound effects at the cellular level, discover strategic fasting techniques for promoting longevity, and learn how to seamlessly integrate mindful living with fasting to unlock the door to a longer, healthier life.

How Fasting Affects Cellular Aging and DNA Repair
At the heart of the remarkable connection between fasting and longevity lies a process known as autophagy, which can be thought of as the cellular "clean-up crew." Autophagy is the body's way of clearing out damaged cells and cellular components, recycling them, and paving the way for new, healthy cells to flourish. Think of it as a rejuvenation process that keeps our cells in optimal working condition.

Fasting, particularly intermittent fasting and extended fasts, is a potent trigger for autophagy. When we abstain from food for an extended period, our bodies enter a state where they must rely on stored energy reserves, primarily in the form of glycogen and fat. During this energy crisis, the body begins to break down and recycle damaged or malfunctioning cellular components through autophagy.

This process isn't just about tidying up; it also extends to DNA repair. As cells undergo autophagy, damaged DNA segments are repaired or replaced, reducing the likelihood of mutations and age-related diseases. It's like having an in-house maintenance team ensuring that the blueprint of your cells remains pristine, preventing the accumulation of genetic errors over time.

But how can you harness the power of fasting to kickstart autophagy and promote cellular rejuvenation? There are several fasting strategies you can explore:

Fasting Strategies for Promoting Longevity
1. Intermittent Fasting: This approach involves cycling between periods of eating and fasting. The most common method is the 16/8, where you fast for 16 hours and eat within an 8-hour window. This routine promotes autophagy and allows your body to repair cellular damage effectively.

2. Extended Fasting: Extended fasting, typically lasting 24 to 48 hours or even longer, is a more profound way to stimulate autophagy and DNA repair. During these extended fasts, your body taps into deeper reserves, initiating a thorough cellular clean-up process.

3. Time-Restricted Eating: If longer fasts seem daunting, you can start with time-restricted eating. Limit your daily

eating window to, for example, 10 hours or less, giving your body an extended fasting period each day.

4. The 5:2 Diet: In this approach, you consume your regular diet for five days of the week and reduce your calorie intake to about 500-600 calories on the remaining two non-consecutive days. This intermittent calorie restriction encourages autophagy while allowing you to maintain a regular eating pattern most of the time.

Now, as promising as these fasting strategies are for promoting longevity, it's essential to approach fasting with mindfulness and caution. Fasting isn't suitable for everyone, and consulting with a healthcare professional before embarking on any fasting regimen is highly recommended, especially if you have underlying medical conditions.

Combining Mindful Living with Fasting for Long-Term Health
While fasting holds immense potential for extending our years on this planet, its true power shines when combined with the principles of mindful living. Mindfulness encourages a heightened awareness of our bodies and an appreciation for the present moment, which can be invaluable when navigating the challenges and rewards of fasting.

Here's how you can combine mindful living with fasting for long-term health:

1. Set Clear Intentions: Begin your fasting journey with a clear understanding of your goals. Whether it's improved longevity, weight management, or enhanced overall health, having a purpose behind your fasting efforts can help you stay committed.

2. Listen to Your Body: Mindful living teaches us to listen to our bodies' cues. During a fast, it's crucial to pay close attention to how you feel. If you experience severe discomfort or dizziness, it may be a sign that your body needs nourishment. Always prioritize safety and well-being.

3. Embrace Gratitude: Mindfulness invites gratitude into our lives. When you break your fast, savor each bite with gratitude for the nourishment it provides. This practice not only enhances your enjoyment of meals but also reinforces a positive relationship with food.

4. Stress Reduction: Mindfulness techniques such as deep breathing and meditation can be incredibly helpful during fasting periods. They assist in managing stress and cravings, making the fasting experience more manageable and enjoyable.

5. Stay Hydrated: Proper hydration is essential during fasting. Mindfully sip water throughout the day to stay hydrated and support your body's detoxification processes.

6. Gradual Implementation: If fasting is new to you, consider starting slowly and gradually increasing the duration of your fasts. Mindfully observe how your body responds and make adjustments accordingly.

As you embark on your journey of combining mindful living with fasting, remember that it's not just about the destination but also the experience along the way. Each moment of mindfulness, each fast, and each nourishing meal is a step toward a longer, healthier life. By weaving together the wisdom of fasting and the art of mindful living, you'll discover the path to not just a longer life, but a richer and more fulfilling one.

7.2 Mindful Living for Aging Gracefully

As we journey through life, the concept of aging gracefully takes on profound meaning. It's not just about looking youthful on the outside; it's about nurturing your mental, emotional, and physical well-being as you traverse the decades. In this subchapter, we'll explore how the principles of mindful living can be your trusted companions on the path to aging gracefully. Let's dive into practical and actionable steps that will empower you to embrace each passing year with purpose and mindfulness.

Mindful Aging Practices for Mental and Emotional Well-being

As we age, it's common to become more critical of ourselves, dwelling on perceived shortcomings or missed opportunities. Mindful living invites you to extend compassion to yourself. Begin by acknowledging your inner critic without judgment. When self-doubt arises, pause and breathe. Ask yourself, "Would I speak to a dear friend this way?" Treat yourself with the same kindness and understanding you'd offer to someone you love. This simple shift in self-talk can significantly enhance your mental and emotional well-being.

Aging gracefully starts with gratitude. Each morning, take a moment to reflect on the blessings in your life. It could be the warmth of the sun on your face, the laughter of a grandchild, or the aroma of your morning coffee. As you cultivate gratitude, you'll find that it has the power to reshape your perspective. It's a gentle reminder of the richness of your life's tapestry. And when challenges arise, gratitude can be your anchor, helping you navigate the storms with resilience.

One of the secrets to staying mentally vibrant as you age is to maintain a curious mind. Embrace new hobbies, interests, and challenges. Take up that instrument you always wanted to learn or explore a foreign language. Engaging in novel experiences keeps your brain agile and adaptable. Additionally, the act of learning fosters a sense of accomplishment and invigorates your mental state.

Mindfulness for Adapting to Physical Changes with Age

Aging often comes with physical changes. Mindful body awareness involves staying attuned to your body's signals without judgment. Regularly check in with yourself. Notice areas of tension or discomfort, and respond with kindness. Engage in gentle stretching or yoga to maintain flexibility.

The goal isn't perfection but rather the nurturing of a harmonious relationship between your mind and body.

As you age, your nutritional needs may shift. Mindful eating can help you make nourishing choices. Pay attention to your body's hunger and fullness cues. Savor each bite, enjoying the flavors and textures. Consider the quality of your food, opting for whole, unprocessed options. Pair mindful eating with mindful movement. Gentle exercises like tai chi or walking in nature can help you stay active and maintain your physical well-being.

Aging gracefully also means embracing change with grace. Your body may not move or function as it once did, and that's okay. Adaptation doesn't imply resignation; it signifies resilience. Modify your daily routines to accommodate your changing needs. Seek out support and resources if necessary. Remember that each phase of life brings its unique gifts and opportunities for growth.

Aging with Purpose and Mindfulness
Aging doesn't diminish your capacity to contribute to the world. In fact, it can deepen it. Take time to reflect on your life's purpose. What passions or causes ignite your spirit? How can you share your wisdom and experience with others? Your sense of purpose will infuse your life with meaning and drive.

As you age, your relationships become even more precious. Nurture deep connections with family and friends. Engage in open and heartfelt conversations. Be present when you spend time with loved ones, cherishing each moment. Meaningful relationships provide emotional sustenance and are a source of joy throughout life.

Aging gracefully isn't about holding onto youth; it's about celebrating the beauty of each age and stage. You've earned every wrinkle and gray hair, each laugh line tells a story of a life well-lived. Embrace your unique journey and the wisdom it has bestowed upon you. Allow your inner light to shine through, illuminating the path for others.

Aging gracefully isn't about defying time but rather about embracing it with mindfulness and purpose. It's about cherishing the moments, nurturing your mental and emotional well-being, adapting with grace, and finding meaning in each day. As you embark on this journey, remember that you are a masterpiece in progress, a testament to the art of living a mindful and purposeful life at any age.

7.3 Fasting and Age-Related Diseases

In the quest for longevity and vibrant health, the art of fasting has emerged as a potent ally. As we journey through life, the inevitability of aging often brings with it a host of age-related diseases and conditions. But what if I told you that fasting could be the key to slowing down this process, allowing us to not just add years to our lives, but life to our years? In this subchapter, we'll delve into fasting's remarkable role in preventing age-related diseases. We'll explore the science behind it, backed by compelling case studies of individuals who have wholeheartedly embraced fasting as a means to extend their vitality.

Fasting's Role in Preventing Age-Related Diseases
Aging is inevitable, but how we age is within our control. Fasting emerges as a formidable ally in our quest for graceful aging. It's not about halting the march of time but rather slowing its impact on our bodies. Fasting, in its various forms, triggers a cascade of biological responses that fortify our defenses against age-related diseases. Here's how it works:

1. Cellular Renewal and Repair: Imagine your body as a complex machine with millions of moving parts. Over time, these parts wear down, accumulate damage, and malfunction. Cellular renewal and repair become critical, and fasting is the mechanic that steps in to fix the wear and tear. During fasting, a process called autophagy is activated. Autophagy literally means 'self-eating,' and it involves your body cleaning up and recycling damaged cells and components. Think of it as a cellular spring cleaning that renews your body from within.

2. Reducing Inflammation: Chronic inflammation is the silent culprit behind numerous age-related diseases, from heart disease to arthritis. Fasting has an anti-inflammatory effect that helps soothe the embers of inflammation in our bodies. By giving our digestive system a break and reducing the intake of inflammatory foods during fasts, we

curb the flames of inflammation and bolster our body's defenses.

3. Insulin Sensitivity: As we age, insulin resistance often creeps in, paving the way for type 2 diabetes and other metabolic disorders. Fasting plays a significant role in improving insulin sensitivity. When you fast, your body becomes more efficient at using insulin, ensuring that blood sugar remains stable. This, in turn, reduces the risk of diabetes and its associated complications.

4. DNA Protection: Our DNA is the blueprint of our existence, and over time, it can suffer damage due to various factors like oxidative stress and environmental toxins. Fasting helps protect our DNA by enhancing the activity of repair mechanisms. It's like having an army of repairmen ready to fix any damage to the blueprint of your life.

5. Cognitive Resilience: Age-related cognitive decline is a concern for many, but fasting may offer a shield against it. Fasting promotes the production of brain-derived neurotrophic factor (BDNF), a protein that supports the growth and maintenance of neurons. This can help protect against neurodegenerative diseases like Alzheimer's.

Now, let's dive into real-life stories, tales of individuals who have not just extended their lifespans but also enriched the quality of their later years through fasting.

Case Studies of Individuals Who Have Embraced Fasting for Longevity

Case Study 1: Maria's Remarkable Transformation

Maria, a 62-year-old retired schoolteacher, was struggling with obesity and high blood pressure. She'd tried various diets without lasting success. However, her introduction to intermittent fasting was a turning point. Maria adopted a 16/8 fasting regimen, fasting for 16 hours and eating during an 8-hour window. Over time, she shed excess weight, and her blood pressure normalized. But that wasn't the most remarkable part of her journey.

Maria's mental clarity and energy levels soared. She felt like she was in her forties again. Her zest for life returned, and she began pursuing hobbies she'd set aside years ago. It's not just about living longer for Maria; it's about living better. Her story is a testament to the rejuvenating power of fasting.

Case Study 2: Robert's Battle Against Diabetes

Robert, a 57-year-old IT professional, was grappling with type 2 diabetes. Despite medication and dietary adjustments, his blood sugar remained stubbornly high. Frustrated with the endless cycle of medications, he turned to fasting as a last resort. He began with periodic extended fasts under medical supervision.

The results were astonishing. Robert's blood sugar levels started to normalize, and he eventually reduced his dependency on medication. He learned to listen to his body and understand hunger cues. Beyond diabetes management, he experienced increased mental clarity and a newfound sense of discipline. Robert's journey shows us that it's never too late to take control of our health and reverse the course of disease.

Case Study 3: Sarah's Journey to Vibrant Aging

Sarah, at 72, is living proof that age is just a number. She embraced fasting and mindful living in her early sixties after witnessing her friends struggle with chronic illnesses. Sarah's approach combines intermittent fasting with a focus on whole, unprocessed foods.

Not only has she maintained a healthy weight, but she's also brimming with vitality. Sarah is an avid traveler, hiker, and artist. Her skin radiates a healthy glow, and her zest for life is contagious. She demonstrates that embracing fasting and mindfulness can lead to a vibrant and fulfilling life well into your golden years.

These case studies illustrate that fasting isn't merely about extending lifespan; it's about enhancing the quality of the years we have. It's about reclaiming our vitality and experiencing life to the fullest. By preventing age-related diseases and rejuvenating our bodies, fasting empowers us to embrace aging as a beautiful and fulfilling journey.

As you embark on your own fasting and longevity adventure, remember that these case studies are not isolated incidents. They represent a growing community of individuals who have harnessed the power of fasting to rewrite their stories of aging. By implementing fasting practices and mindful living techniques, you too can pave the way for a healthier, more vibrant, and fulfilling future.

Chapter 8: Mindful Stress Management Techniques

8.1 Understanding Stress and Its Impact on Health

Stress. It's a word we all know too well. In the fast-paced, demanding world we live in, stress seems to be a constant companion. We often wear it like a badge of honor, a sign that we're pushing ourselves to our limits. But the truth is, chronic stress can take a toll on our physical and mental well-being in ways we may not even realize.

The Science of Stress and Its Physical Effects

Let's begin by peeling back the layers and understanding what stress really is, beyond just the feeling of tension and anxiety. Stress is a physiological response triggered by our body's ancient "fight or flight" system. When faced with a perceived threat, whether it's a tight deadline at work, a challenging personal relationship, or financial worries, our body releases a surge of stress hormones, primarily cortisol and adrenaline.

These stress hormones prepare our body to respond to the threat. Our heart rate increases, our muscles tense, and our senses become sharper. This response served our ancestors well when facing physical dangers like wild animals, but in today's world, our stressors are often more abstract and ongoing.

The problem arises when our bodies remain in this heightened state of alertness for extended periods. Chronic stress can lead to a cascade of physical effects, including:

- Cardiovascular Issues: Prolonged stress can contribute to high blood pressure, increasing the risk of heart disease and stroke. The constant strain on the heart takes a toll over time.

- Digestive Problems: Stress can disrupt the digestive system, leading to issues such as irritable bowel syndrome (IBS), acid reflux, and even ulcers. It's no coincidence that we often say we have a "knot in our stomach" when stressed.

- Weakened Immune System: Stress suppresses the immune system, making us more susceptible to infections and illnesses. It's as if chronic stress pries open the door for pathogens to enter.

- Mental Health Challenges: Beyond physical health, stress plays a significant role in mental health disorders such as anxiety and depression. The constant wear and tear on our mental resilience can erode our emotional well-being.

Understanding the physiological basis of stress is the first step in combating it. It's not merely a mental state but a physical response with far-reaching consequences. Recognizing that chronic stress isn't something to be ignored is essential.

Identifying Sources of Stress in Daily Life

Now that we grasp the science behind stress, the next step is to identify the sources of stress in our daily lives. This can be a profoundly personal process because what causes stress for one person may not affect another in the same way.

Start by taking a moment to reflect on your daily routines and activities. What situations or responsibilities tend to make you feel overwhelmed, anxious, or irritable? These might be:

- Work Pressure: The demands of your job, tight deadlines, and the expectation to perform at your peak can create tremendous stress.

- Relationship Struggles: Conflicts with family members, friends, or romantic partners can be major sources of stress. Interpersonal dynamics can be complex and emotionally draining.

- Financial Worries: Money concerns, such as debt, bills, or uncertainty about the future, can be a constant source of anxiety.

- Health Challenges: If you're dealing with a chronic illness or health issues, the stress of managing your condition can be significant.

- Overcommitment: Trying to do too much in too little time can leave you feeling perpetually rushed and stressed.

- Life Transitions: Major life changes like moving, changing jobs, or starting a family can be exciting but also extremely stressful.

Remember, it's not about comparing your stressors to others' but recognizing the impact they have on your own well-being. Stress can accumulate over time, so even seemingly small stressors can take a toll if they're persistent.

The Connection Between Stress and Disease
Here's where the stakes get higher. Stress isn't just an uncomfortable feeling; it's a significant contributor to many chronic diseases. The connection between stress and disease is not a matter of coincidence; it's firmly grounded in scientific research.

Chronic stress, with its constant release of stress hormones, can create the perfect conditions for disease to take hold and thrive. Here are some of the ways stress and disease are intertwined:

- Inflammation: Chronic stress triggers inflammation in the body, which is linked to a host of diseases, including cardiovascular disease, diabetes, and even cancer.

- Weakened Immunity: As mentioned earlier, stress suppresses the immune system, making us more susceptible to infections and illnesses.

- Metabolic Changes: Stress can lead to unhealthy eating habits and weight gain, increasing the risk of conditions like obesity and type 2 diabetes.

- Mental Health: The relationship between stress and mental health disorders is well-established. Chronic stress can contribute to anxiety, depression, and other mood disorders.

- Cardiovascular Impact: Stress can raise blood pressure, which is a major risk factor for heart disease. It can also lead to unhealthy habits like smoking or excessive drinking, further increasing the risk.

Recognizing the connection between stress and disease isn't about adding more worry to your plate but empowering yourself to take action. Stress isn't a given; it's something you can manage and mitigate. In the following subchapters, we'll delve into practical and actionable steps to help you do just that.

8.2 Mindful Techniques for Stress Reduction

Stress is an omnipresent part of modern life. From work pressures to personal challenges, it can sometimes feel overwhelming. But here's the good news: you have the power to manage and even conquer stress through mindful living techniques. In this subchapter, we'll explore some practical and actionable steps that will help you build your stress resilience toolkit.

Mindful Meditation for Stress Relief
Meditation is a time-tested practice that can work wonders when it comes to stress management. It's not about sitting cross-legged for hours or emptying your mind of all thoughts. Instead, it's about finding a few moments each day to quiet your mind, connect with your breath, and create a sense of inner calm.

Actionable Step 1: Find Your Zen Zone

Choose a quiet space where you won't be disturbed. Sit comfortably in a chair or on the floor, with your back straight and your hands resting on your lap. Close your eyes if you feel comfortable doing so.

Actionable Step 2: Breathe Deeply and Mindfully

Begin to focus on your breath. Inhale slowly and deeply through your nose, counting to four as you do. Feel the air filling your lungs and expanding your chest. Now, exhale slowly through your mouth, counting to six as you release the breath. As you breathe, notice the rise and fall of your abdomen with each inhale and exhale.

Actionable Step 3: Embrace the Present Moment

Thoughts will inevitably drift into your mind as you meditate. That's okay; it's perfectly normal. The key is not to engage with these thoughts. Instead, gently acknowledge them and let them float away like leaves on a stream. Bring your attention back to your breath. This simple act of refocusing is a core aspect of mindfulness.

Actionable Step 4: Start Small and Build

If you're new to meditation, don't expect to meditate for an hour right away. Start with just five minutes each day and gradually increase the duration as you become more comfortable. Consistency is more important than the duration of your practice.

Meditation isn't a quick fix, but with regular practice, it can help you build resilience to stress. As you become more skilled at redirecting your focus, you'll find that stressors have less power to rattle you.

Mindful Breathing Exercises and Their Benefits

Breathing is one of the most accessible and effective tools for managing stress. Our breath is intimately connected to our emotions, and by learning to control our breath, we can gain greater control over our stress response.

Actionable Step 1: The 4-7-8 Breath

This simple technique is a game-changer when it comes to stress reduction. Start by sitting or lying down in a comfortable position. Close your eyes and take a deep breath in through your nose for a count of four. Hold your breath for a count of seven. Finally, exhale slowly and completely through your mouth for a count of eight. Repeat this cycle four times.

Actionable Step 2: Box Breathing

Box breathing is another excellent technique that can help you regain control over your stress response. Imagine drawing the sides of a square. As you do, inhale for a count of four, hold your breath for a count of four, exhale for a count of four, and hold your breath again for a count of four. Repeat this process for several cycles.

Actionable Step 3: Breath Awareness

Simply paying attention to your breath as it is, without trying to control it, can be a powerful stress-reduction technique. Find a quiet place to sit or lie down. Close your eyes and bring your attention to your breath. Notice the sensation of the breath as it enters and leaves your body. Is it cool or warm? Is it shallow or deep? Does it have a rhythm? Stay with this awareness for a few minutes.

Mindfulness-Based Stress Reduction (MBSR) Techniques

MBSR is a structured program developed by Dr. Jon Kabat-Zinn that combines mindfulness meditation and yoga to reduce stress and enhance well-being. While MBSR is typically taught in a group setting over an eight-week period, you can incorporate some of its principles into your daily life.

Actionable Step 1: The Body Scan Meditation

The body scan is a fundamental practice in MBSR. Lie down in a comfortable position and close your eyes. Starting at the top of your head, bring your awareness to each part of your body, moving slowly downward. Notice any areas of tension or discomfort, and consciously release them with your breath.

Actionable Step 2: Mindful Eating

Eating mindfully is an excellent way to reduce stress and improve your relationship with food. Choose a meal or snack and commit to eating it without distractions. Pay close attention to the colors, textures, and flavors of your food. Chew slowly and savor each bite. Notice how your body feels as you eat. Are you hungry or full? Are there any emotions connected to this meal?

Actionable Step 3: Mindful Walking

Walking can be a mindfulness practice when done with intention. Take a walk outdoors and focus on the sensations of movement. Feel your feet lifting off the ground and making contact again. Notice the air on your skin and the sounds around you. If your mind wanders to stressful thoughts, gently bring your attention back to the present moment.

Incorporating MBSR techniques into your life can provide a structured and effective way to manage stress. While it may take time to fully integrate these practices, the benefits in terms of reduced stress and increased well-being are well worth the effort.

Stress is a part of life, but it doesn't have to overwhelm you. By incorporating mindful techniques like meditation, breathing exercises, and MBSR principles into your daily routine, you can build your stress resilience and cultivate a greater sense of calm and balance. Remember that these practices take time to develop, so be patient with yourself and celebrate each step forward in your journey toward stress management and overall well-being.

8.3 Mindful Living as a Stress-Resilience Tool

Stress has become an unwelcome companion in our modern lives. Whether it's the demands of work, family responsibilities, or the never-ending buzz of technology, stress seems to lurk around every corner. But there's a powerful antidote to this stress epidemic, and it's called mindful living. In this subchapter, we'll dive deep into the world of mindful living as a stress-resilience tool. You'll discover how mindfulness can not only help you manage stress but also build the kind of resilience that allows you to navigate life's challenges with grace and composure.

How Mindful Living Builds Stress Resilience

Imagine your mind as a calm lake, undisturbed by the ripples of stress. This is the essence of stress resilience, and mindfulness is the stone that gently drops into the water, creating those serene ripples. How does it work?

1. Presence in the Moment: Mindfulness is all about being fully present in the moment. When you practice mindfulness, you train your mind to focus on what's happening right now, rather than worrying about the past or future. This presence allows you to confront stressors head-on, without being overwhelmed.

2. Embracing Acceptance: Mindfulness teaches us to accept things as they are, without judgment. When you can accept your circumstances, even if they're stressful, it becomes easier to deal with them. You're no longer fighting against reality but flowing with it.

3. Emotional Regulation: Mindful living equips you with the tools to regulate your emotions. Instead of reacting impulsively to stress, you can observe your emotional responses and choose how to respond. This emotional intelligence is a vital aspect of stress resilience.

Creating a Mindful Environment for Reducing Stress
Mindfulness isn't just a practice you engage in; it's a way of life. Creating a mindful environment can significantly contribute to reducing stress in your daily life. Here's how to do it:

1. Simplify Your Space: Start by decluttering your physical space. A cluttered environment often leads to a cluttered mind. Create a clean, organized space that promotes a sense of calm and clarity.

2. Digital Detox: Our screens bombard us with information and notifications, adding to our stress levels. Consider implementing regular digital detoxes, where you disconnect from devices and reconnect with the real world.

3. Nature Connection: Nature has a remarkable ability to soothe the soul. Spend time outdoors, whether it's a walk in the park, a hike in the woods, or simply sitting in your backyard. Nature provides a serene backdrop for mindfulness.

4. Mindful Design: Pay attention to the design and aesthetics of your surroundings. Colors, lighting, and textures can influence your mood. Choose elements that promote tranquility and comfort.

Mindfulness for Coping with Chronic Stressors

Chronic stressors, those long-term challenges that seem to have no end in sight, can take a toll on your well-being. Mindfulness offers valuable tools for coping with these persistent stressors:

1. Daily Mindfulness Practice: Establish a daily mindfulness practice, even if it's just for a few minutes. This regularity builds your resilience over time, helping you better cope with chronic stressors.

2. Mindful Breathing: Your breath is always with you, serving as a anchor to the present moment. When faced with chronic stress, take a moment to focus on your breath. Inhale deeply, exhale slowly, and let go of tension.

3. Mindful Problem-Solving: Instead of ruminating on the problem, mindfully engage in problem-solving. Break it down into smaller, manageable steps, and approach it one step at a time. This approach reduces overwhelm.

4. Self-Compassion: Chronic stress can lead to self-criticism. Practice self-compassion by treating yourself with the same kindness and understanding you would offer to a friend facing a similar situation.

5. Seek Support: Don't hesitate to seek support from a therapist or counselor if chronic stress becomes too much to handle alone. Mindfulness can be a valuable complement to professional help.

Mindful Living in Action

Let's put mindful living into action with a practical exercise. Take a moment to find a comfortable seat. Close your eyes if that feels comfortable for you; otherwise, just soften your gaze.

Begin by taking a deep breath in, allowing your lungs to fill completely, and then exhale slowly and completely. As you breathe, bring your attention to the sensations in your body. Notice any areas of tension or discomfort.

Now, imagine your body relaxing with each breath. Imagine that tension melting away, like ice turning into water. Feel the soothing rhythm of your breath, the rise and fall of your chest or abdomen.

As you continue to breathe mindfully, bring your awareness to any thoughts or worries that may be causing you stress. Don't judge them or try to push them away. Simply acknowledge their presence, like clouds passing in the sky.

With each breath, imagine those thoughts floating away, leaving behind a clear, peaceful sky. Allow yourself to fully inhabit this moment of calm and clarity.

When you're ready, slowly open your eyes and return to your surroundings. You've just experienced a taste of mindful living in action. This practice can be a lifeline during times of stress, helping you find peace and resilience in the midst of life's challenges.

Incorporate mindfulness into your daily life, and you'll discover that stress no longer has the same grip on you. With each mindful breath, you build the resilience to face whatever comes your way with poise and presence. It's a transformative journey, and you're well on your way to mastering it.

Chapter 9: Fasting and Chronic Disease Prevention

9.1 Fasting and Insulin Sensitivity

Fasting has emerged as a powerful tool in the fight against chronic diseases, and one of its most remarkable effects is on insulin sensitivity. Insulin sensitivity is the body's ability to respond effectively to insulin, a hormone that regulates blood sugar levels. When your body becomes resistant to insulin, it struggles to control blood sugar, increasing the risk of type 2 diabetes and other chronic health issues. But fret not, because fasting can be a game-changer in this arena. In this subchapter, we'll dive deep into how fasting enhances insulin sensitivity, how it can prevent and manage type 2 diabetes, and how you can tailor your fasting approach to take control of your insulin levels.

Fasting's Role in Improving Insulin Sensitivity

The concept of fasting improving insulin sensitivity may seem counterintuitive at first. After all, isn't fasting about not eating? How can that help with blood sugar regulation? The magic lies in the body's adaptive response to fasting.

During fasting periods, when you abstain from food for a set duration, your body taps into its energy reserves, particularly stored glucose (glycogen) and fat. As this happens, your insulin levels drop significantly. This break from constantly elevated insulin levels gives your cells a chance to "reset" and become more receptive to insulin when it returns.

Think of it as a reset button for your metabolism. Your cells become more efficient at taking in glucose from your bloodstream, reducing the need for higher insulin levels to manage blood sugar. This improved sensitivity to insulin means your body can use glucose more effectively, preventing blood sugar spikes and subsequent crashes.

Fasting's impact on insulin sensitivity doesn't stop there. It also helps reduce inflammation in the body. Chronic inflammation can contribute to insulin resistance, so by reducing inflammation through fasting, you're indirectly improving insulin sensitivity.

But how does this translate into real-world benefits? Let's explore...

Using Fasting to Prevent and Manage Type 2 Diabetes

Type 2 diabetes is a condition characterized by insulin resistance. People with this condition have trouble using insulin effectively, leading to high blood sugar levels. If left uncontrolled, it can lead to serious health complications.

Fasting offers a promising approach to preventing and managing type 2 diabetes. Here's how:

1. Prevention: If you're at risk of developing type 2 diabetes due to family history or lifestyle factors, fasting can be a proactive strategy. By regularly incorporating fasting periods into your routine, you can enhance your insulin

sensitivity and reduce the likelihood of developing diabetes in the first place.

2. Management: For those already diagnosed with type 2 diabetes, fasting can be an effective complementary approach to managing the condition. It helps control blood sugar levels by improving insulin sensitivity. However, it's crucial to work closely with your healthcare provider to adjust medications and insulin dosages as needed while fasting safely.

Personalized Fasting Plans for Insulin Control
Now that you understand the benefits of fasting for insulin sensitivity, let's talk about how to incorporate fasting into your life in a personalized way. Remember, there's no one-size-fits-all approach to fasting, and it's essential to find a fasting routine that suits your individual needs and preferences.

1. Intermittent Fasting (IF): This popular fasting method involves cycling between periods of eating and fasting. You can start with a simple 16/8 schedule, where you fast for 16 hours and eat during an 8-hour window. Gradually, you can extend your fasting window to 18 or 20 hours if your body responds well. IF is an excellent choice for improving insulin sensitivity because it allows your body to reset between meals.

2. Extended Fasts: Longer fasting periods, such as 24 hours or more, can be done occasionally or as part of a more extended fasting regimen. Extended fasts provide a more

profound reset for your insulin sensitivity and can be particularly helpful for those at high risk of type 2 diabetes or looking to manage the condition.

3. Alternate-Day Fasting: This approach involves alternating between fasting days and regular eating days. It can be effective for some people in improving insulin sensitivity, but it may be more challenging to maintain in the long term.

4. Consult with a Healthcare Professional: Before embarking on any fasting regimen, especially if you have diabetes or other underlying health conditions, it's crucial to consult with a healthcare professional. They can help you create a personalized fasting plan that aligns with your health goals and ensures your safety.

5. Monitor Your Blood Sugar: Whether you're at risk of diabetes or managing the condition, regularly monitoring your blood sugar levels is essential. Keep a record of your readings and share them with your healthcare provider. This information will help tailor your fasting plan to your specific needs.

Incorporating fasting into your life can be a powerful strategy for improving insulin sensitivity, preventing type 2 diabetes, and managing the condition if you already have it. Remember that fasting is a lifestyle choice and should be approached mindfully. It's not about deprivation but about optimizing your health and well-being.

9.2 Fasting for Heart Health

Our heart, that steadfast organ pumping life through our veins, is at the core of our vitality. It's the rhythmic drum that keeps us going, and yet, it's also a fragile instrument susceptible to wear and tear over time. Cardiovascular diseases, including heart attacks and strokes, have long been the leading cause of death worldwide. The good news is that we hold the keys to protect this vital organ through fasting and mindful living.

How Fasting Supports Cardiovascular Health

Let's dive right into it. How can fasting, the practice of abstaining from food for a certain period, possibly support cardiovascular health? The answer lies in the profound impact fasting has on your body's inner workings.

When you fast, especially during extended fasts, your body undergoes a series of remarkable changes. One of the most striking is the reduction in blood pressure. High blood pressure, or hypertension, is a silent assassin responsible for numerous heart-related problems. Fasting helps to bring down those numbers, giving your heart a much-needed respite.

Moreover, fasting is like a spring cleaning for your arteries. It clears out the plaque buildup that narrows them, making it harder for blood to flow. Imagine fasting as a gentle stream of water gradually eroding away the obstacles in its path. This unclogs your arteries, allowing for improved circulation and reducing the risk of heart disease.

But it's not just about what fasting does; it's also about what it doesn't do. During fasting periods, your body enters a state called autophagy, where it starts to self-repair. Think of it as your body's maintenance mode. It gets rid of damaged cells and proteins, making way for healthier ones. This process extends to your heart muscles, promoting cardiovascular resilience.

Mindful Living for Cholesterol Control

Cholesterol is a buzzword often associated with heart problems, but not all cholesterol is bad. There's a good kind, HDL (high-density lipoprotein), which works like a scavenger, cleaning up excess cholesterol from your bloodstream. Then there's LDL (low-density lipoprotein), the one we need to keep in check. High levels of LDL cholesterol can lead to plaque buildup in your arteries.

Enter mindful living as a vital player in this heart-protective game. Mindful eating, in particular, is a powerful tool. When you eat mindfully, you become more aware of the quality of the food you consume. It's not just about calories; it's about nourishing your body with the right nutrients.

Choose foods that support heart health. Think of colorful fruits and vegetables, whole grains, and lean proteins. These choices can help lower your LDL cholesterol levels and reduce your risk of heart disease.

Mindful eating also encourages portion control. Overeating, especially when it involves high-calorie, high-fat foods, can contribute to obesity and increased cholesterol levels. Slowing down and savoring each bite allows your body to register fullness, preventing you from overindulging.

Mindful Living Practices for Heart Disease Prevention

Prevention is the cornerstone of a healthy heart. Instead of waiting for problems to arise, why not embrace mindful living practices that fortify your heart and keep it resilient? Here's a practical approach:

Mindful Eating: When you consume your meals mindfully, you're not just feeding your body; you're nourishing your heart. Savor each bite, chew slowly, and pay attention to the flavors and textures. This not only makes your meals more enjoyable but also helps you make healthier food choices.

Regular Exercise: Mindful movement, such as yoga or tai chi, is an excellent choice for heart health. These practices not only keep you physically active but also enhance your mind-body connection. Aim for at least 150 minutes of moderate-intensity aerobic activity every week.

Stress Management: Stress can be a silent heartbreaker. Incorporate mindfulness meditation into your daily routine. Even just a few minutes of deep breathing exercises can go a long way in reducing stress and promoting heart health.

Quality Sleep: Don't underestimate the power of sleep. A well-rested body is better equipped to handle the demands of daily life, including those on your heart. Create a sleep-conducive environment, maintain a regular sleep schedule, and unwind before bedtime.

Regular Check-ups: Mindful living involves being proactive about your health. Schedule regular check-ups with your healthcare provider to monitor your heart health. Early detection and intervention can be lifesaving.

Real-Life Success Stories of Individuals Who Reversed Heart Disease with Fasting

You might be wondering, "Does fasting really work for heart disease?" The answer lies in the inspiring journeys of individuals who have faced the daunting prospect of heart disease and emerged victorious through fasting and mindful living.

Meet Annie, a vibrant 45-year-old woman who was diagnosed with high blood pressure and elevated cholesterol levels. Fearing the potential consequences, she decided to take control of her health. Annie began incorporating intermittent fasting into her routine, along with a mindful approach to her diet.

She started by eliminating processed foods and prioritizing heart-healthy choices like fruits, vegetables, whole grains, and lean proteins. As a result, her LDL cholesterol levels began to decrease, and her blood pressure returned to a healthy range. Annie 's transformation wasn't just physical; she felt more energetic and mentally focused than ever before.

Then there's William, a 55-year-old man with a family history of heart disease. Determined not to follow in his family's footsteps, he embarked on a journey of intermittent fasting. With guidance from his healthcare provider and the support of a mindful living community, William started fasting for 16 hours each day, allowing his body to tap into its fat stores and improve insulin sensitivity.

After several months, William's weight dropped, and his cholesterol levels improved significantly. His heart health began to mirror the heart health of individuals without a family history of heart disease. William 's story serves as a testament to the transformative power of fasting and mindful living in the prevention of heart disease.

These real-life success stories remind us that the path to heart health is not unattainable. By embracing fasting and mindful living practices, you can take charge of your cardiovascular well-being and, like Annie and William, rewrite the narrative of your heart's journey.

The connection between fasting and heart health is profound, and when coupled with mindful living practices, it becomes a formidable force in the prevention and reversal of heart disease. By understanding how fasting supports cardiovascular health, adopting mindful eating habits, and incorporating mindful living practices, you too can embark on a journey towards a heart-healthy and vibrant life. The real-life success stories of individuals who've transformed their heart health through these practices are a testament to the potential that lies within each of us to nurture and protect our most vital organ—the heart.

9.3 Fasting and Cancer Prevention

In our journey to explore the profound effects of fasting on chronic disease prevention, we arrive at a critical juncture - the link between fasting and cancer prevention. Cancer, an insidious and life-altering disease, touches the lives of countless individuals and their families. But here's the thing: while genetics play a role, our lifestyle choices, including what and when we eat, can significantly influence our susceptibility to cancer. In this subchapter, we'll dive deep into the science-backed connection between fasting and cancer prevention, explore how mindful living can fortify us against this formidable foe, and provide you with personalized fasting and lifestyle strategies that can potentially reduce your risk of cancer.

The Link Between Fasting and Cancer Prevention

Let's get straight to the heart of the matter. Can fasting really help prevent cancer? The short answer is yes, and here's why:

Cancer cells thrive in an environment that's fueled by a constant supply of nutrients, especially glucose. When we fast, we temporarily cut off this supply, making it challenging for cancer cells to grow and divide. In fact, fasting has been shown to induce a state known as autophagy, a cellular cleaning process, which can selectively eliminate damaged cells, including those that could become cancerous.

Moreover, fasting reduces inflammation, a key driver of cancer development. Chronic inflammation can create a conducive environment for cancer to flourish. Fasting, through its anti-inflammatory effects, helps create a hostile terrain for potential cancer cells.

But here's the exciting part: fasting doesn't just hinder cancer progression; it may also help prevent its onset. Some studies suggest that intermittent fasting and periodic extended fasts can promote apoptosis, which is the programmed death of damaged or harmful cells, including precancerous ones.

Mindful Living for Cancer Resilience
While fasting provides a formidable shield against cancer, it's not the only player in the game. Mindful living complements fasting in creating a holistic strategy to protect your body from cancer's clutches.

Mindfulness is about tuning into your body, emotions, and environment. When it comes to cancer prevention, this heightened awareness can make all the difference. Here's how:

Firstly, mindfulness helps you make informed dietary choices. You become attuned to your body's signals, making it easier to choose foods that support health and steer clear of those that may promote cancer. You're less likely to indulge in processed, sugary, and inflammatory foods.

Secondly, mindfulness reduces stress. Chronic stress suppresses your immune system, making you more vulnerable to diseases, including cancer. Mindfulness techniques like meditation and deep breathing can counteract stress's harmful effects, bolstering your body's defense against cancer.

Thirdly, mindfulness fosters a sense of purpose and positivity. A positive outlook on life can boost your immune system and encourage healthier behaviors. When you engage in mindful living, you're more likely to adopt habits that promote overall well-being, including cancer prevention.

Personalized Fasting and Lifestyle Strategies for Cancer Prevention

Now, let's talk about actionable steps you can take to leverage the power of fasting and mindfulness for cancer prevention. Remember, everyone is unique, so it's essential to tailor your approach to your individual needs and circumstances.

1. Consult a Healthcare Professional: Before embarking on any fasting regimen, consult your healthcare provider, especially if you have any underlying health conditions or are currently undergoing cancer treatment.

2. Start with Intermittent Fasting: Begin with intermittent fasting, which involves cycling between periods of eating and fasting. A popular method is the 16/8, where you fast for 16 hours and eat within an 8-hour window. This approach can be easier to integrate into your daily routine.

3. Gradually Extend Fasting Periods: If you're comfortable with intermittent fasting, consider incorporating longer fasting periods. Options include the 5:2 method (eating normally for five days and limiting calorie intake for two non-consecutive days) or a 24-hour fast once a week.

4. Mindful Eating: Pay attention to what you eat when you break your fast. Opt for a balanced, plant-based diet rich in colorful fruits and vegetables, which are loaded with cancer-fighting antioxidants. Minimize processed foods, sugary drinks, and red meat.

5. Mindful Stress Reduction: Incorporate mindfulness practices into your daily routine to manage stress effectively. Whether it's a short morning meditation, a calming breathing exercise before bed, or regular mindfulness breaks throughout the day, find what works best for you.

6. Stay Physically Active: Engage in regular physical activity, as it complements your cancer prevention efforts. Mindful movement, such as yoga or tai chi, can be particularly beneficial, as it combines exercise with stress reduction techniques.

7. Regular Screenings and Check-ups: Continue to attend regular cancer screenings and health check-ups. Fasting and

mindfulness are complementary strategies, not substitutes for conventional medical care.

8. Keep a Journal: Maintain a journal to track your fasting and mindful living journey. Note how you feel physically and emotionally, any challenges you encounter, and your achievements. This self-awareness can motivate and guide you along the way.

Cancer prevention is a battlefield, and fasting and mindfulness are potent allies to have by your side. By understanding the link between fasting and cancer prevention, embracing mindful living, and personalizing your fasting and lifestyle strategies, you're taking proactive steps to safeguard your health. Remember, small changes can lead to significant outcomes, and your commitment to a mindful, fasting lifestyle may be your most potent defense against the shadow of cancer.

9.4 Fasting for Hormone-Related Conditions

Hormones are the body's messengers, orchestrating everything from our mood to our metabolism. Hormonal imbalances, especially among women with conditions like Polycystic Ovary Syndrome (PCOS), and even among men, can lead to a myriad of health issues. The good news is that fasting can play a significant role in restoring hormonal balance and enhancing overall well-being.

Fasting for PCOS and Hormonal Disorders in Women

Polycystic Ovary Syndrome, commonly known as PCOS, affects millions of women worldwide. It's a hormonal disorder characterized by irregular periods, ovarian cysts, and imbalances in hormones like insulin and androgens. PCOS can lead to weight gain, infertility, and an increased risk of diabetes and heart disease. For women grappling with PCOS, fasting offers a beacon of hope.

1. Intermittent Fasting and PCOS: Intermittent fasting, a pattern of eating that alternates between periods of fasting and eating, has shown promise in managing PCOS. During the fasting window, insulin sensitivity improves, helping to regulate blood sugar levels and reduce the risk of diabetes.

2. The Role of Autophagy: Autophagy, the body's natural cellular cleaning process, is heightened during fasting. This can be particularly beneficial for women with PCOS, as it helps the body remove damaged cells and may contribute to hormone regulation.

3. Mindful Eating: Beyond fasting, mindful eating practices are essential for managing PCOS. Paying attention to food choices and eating mindfully can help women with PCOS make healthier choices, reduce overeating, and manage their weight.

Balancing Hormones through Fasting and Mindful Nutrition

Hormonal imbalances aren't limited to PCOS; they can affect women and men of all ages. Fasting can be a potent tool to bring these hormones back into equilibrium, but it should be combined with mindful nutrition for maximum effectiveness.

1. Hormone Sensitivity: Fasting enhances hormone sensitivity, meaning your body can respond more effectively to the hormonal signals it receives. This can help regulate insulin, thyroid hormones, and sex hormones.

2. Strategic Nutrient Timing: Pairing fasting with strategic nutrient timing can be particularly effective. For instance, breaking your fast with nutrient-dense foods like leafy greens, lean proteins, and healthy fats can support hormonal health.

3. Omega-3 Fatty Acids: Omega-3 fatty acids, found in foods like fatty fish, flaxseeds, and walnuts, can help reduce inflammation and support hormonal balance. Including these in your diet during eating windows can be advantageous.

4. Hydration: Proper hydration is key to hormonal balance. Water helps transport hormones throughout the body, so staying well-hydrated is crucial.

Fasting Strategies for Men's Hormonal Health

Hormonal health is not solely a concern for women; men also face hormonal challenges that can impact their well-being. Fasting strategies can be tailored to address these concerns.

1. Testosterone Optimization: Testosterone, the primary male sex hormone, plays a vital role in muscle growth, mood, and libido. Fasting, combined with strength training, can help optimize testosterone levels.

2. Cortisol Regulation: Chronic stress can lead to elevated cortisol levels, which can negatively impact testosterone and overall health. Intermittent fasting and mindful stress management techniques work in synergy to regulate cortisol.

3. Protein Intake: Adequate protein intake is crucial for maintaining muscle mass and hormonal health. During eating windows, focus on high-quality protein sources like lean meats, fish, and plant-based options like tofu and legumes.

4. Healthy Fats: Incorporating healthy fats, such as avocados, nuts, and olive oil, into your diet can support hormonal balance. These fats are essential for the production of hormones.

5. Sleep Quality: Don't underestimate the importance of sleep. Poor sleep can disrupt hormone production and regulation. Prioritize good sleep hygiene practices to optimize hormonal health.

Remember, fasting is a powerful tool, but it should be approached with caution, especially if you have underlying health conditions. Consulting with a healthcare professional or a registered dietitian who specializes in hormonal health is a wise step to take.

Fasting offers a holistic approach to hormonal balance. It can help women with PCOS manage their condition and support overall hormonal health for both men and women. When combined with mindful nutrition and lifestyle choices, fasting becomes a transformative force for preventing and managing hormone-related conditions. Embrace these strategies and take charge of your hormonal health today.

9.5 Fasting for Gastrointestinal Disorders

When it comes to our overall well-being, the health of our gastrointestinal (GI) system plays a pivotal role. Digestive issues like Irritable Bowel Syndrome (IBS) and Gastroesophageal Reflux Disease (GERD) can disrupt our daily lives and even lead to long-term health complications. But the good news is that fasting, when combined with mindful eating, can be a powerful tool for managing and alleviating these conditions. In this subchapter, we'll delve into the world of fasting as a means to promote gut health and explore mindful eating strategies that can transform your digestive experience.

Fasting for Digestive Disorders like IBS and GERD

Digestive disorders like IBS and GERD can significantly disrupt daily life, making the simplest meals feel like a minefield. If you're one of the many who struggle with these conditions, you know the pain, discomfort, and frustration they bring.

Now, you may be wondering how fasting could possibly help with these conditions. Isn't skipping meals a recipe for disaster when you have a sensitive stomach? The answer lies in the profound effects of fasting on your digestive system.

1. Rest for Your Digestive Tract: When you fast, you give your gastrointestinal tract a well-deserved break. This temporary respite allows it to heal, repair, and reset. For individuals with IBS and GERD, this can mean reduced inflammation and less irritation.

2. Balancing Gut Bacteria: Fasting can promote a healthier balance of gut bacteria. An imbalanced gut microbiome is often a factor in digestive disorders. By allowing beneficial bacteria to thrive, fasting can contribute to a happier gut.

3. Reducing Food Triggers: With fasting, you're naturally avoiding certain foods for a period. This can be especially helpful if you suspect specific food triggers exacerbate your symptoms. By eliminating these triggers during fasting periods, you may experience less discomfort.

4. Mindful Timing: Mindful fasting means you're choosing when and how to fast wisely. You'll work with your body's natural rhythms and consider how fasting aligns with your

daily routine. This can be particularly beneficial for individuals with IBS, as irregular eating patterns can trigger symptoms.

But remember, fasting for digestive disorders should always be approached with caution and under the guidance of a healthcare professional. Every individual is unique, and what works for one may not work for another.

Mindful Eating Strategies for Better Digestion

Now that we've touched on the potential benefits of fasting, let's talk about what happens when you do eat. Mindful eating is your secret weapon in the battle against gastrointestinal disorders.

1: Slow Down and Savor

One of the core principles of mindful eating is slowing down. In our fast-paced world, it's easy to inhale a meal in a matter of minutes. But for those with digestive issues, rushing through meals can spell trouble.

Instead, take your time. Savor each bite, and chew your food thoroughly. This not only aids digestion but also allows you to enjoy your meal fully. When you eat slowly and mindfully, you're less likely to overeat, a common trigger for IBS symptoms.

2: Pay Attention to Food Choices

What you eat matters, especially when you have a sensitive gut. It's essential to identify trigger foods that worsen your symptoms. Common culprits include spicy foods, caffeine, and dairy products.

Keep a food diary to track your meals and note any adverse reactions. This will help you pinpoint specific foods that might be causing trouble. Remember, what triggers one person's symptoms may not affect another, so your journey to better digestive health is highly personalized.

3: Portion Control and Smaller, Frequent Meals

Rather than three large meals a day, consider eating smaller, more frequent meals. This approach can be particularly beneficial for individuals with GERD. Smaller meals place less strain on your stomach and may help prevent acid reflux episodes.

Moreover, when you consume smaller portions, you're less likely to experience the bloating and discomfort often associated with IBS.

Success Stories of Individuals Who Improved Their Gut Health with Fasting and Mindfulness

The proof is in the pudding, as they say. Many individuals have successfully managed their IBS and GERD by

incorporating fasting and mindful eating into their lives.
Let's look at a couple of inspiring success stories:

Anna's Journey to IBS Relief

Anna had battled IBS for years. The unpredictable nature of
her symptoms made it challenging to maintain a social life
and enjoy her favorite foods. Determined to find relief, she
decided to give intermittent fasting a try.

Anna started with a 16/8 fasting schedule, which meant
fasting for 16 hours and eating during an 8-hour window.
During her fasting period, she noticed a significant
reduction in bloating and cramping. She also became more
mindful of her food choices and began avoiding trigger
foods.

Over time, Anna's IBS symptoms became more
manageable. She even ventured into occasional 24-hour
fasts and experienced further improvements. Today, she
swears by the combination of fasting and mindful eating for
keeping her IBS in check.

Mark's Journey to GERD Remission

Mark had struggled with GERD for years. He relied heavily
on medications to manage his symptoms, but the relief was
temporary, and the side effects were bothersome. Desperate
for a more sustainable solution, he delved into the world of
fasting and mindful eating.

Mark began with shorter fasting windows, gradually increasing the duration as his body adapted. He also paid close attention to his food choices, avoiding spicy and acidic foods that triggered his reflux. Mark noticed a remarkable improvement in his GERD symptoms within weeks.

As his journey continued, Mark was able to reduce his medication under the guidance of his healthcare provider. Today, he rarely experiences acid reflux, and he attributes his improved gut health to fasting and mindful eating.

Fasting and mindful eating can be powerful tools in the fight against gastrointestinal disorders like IBS and GERD. While these approaches may not provide an instant cure, they offer a path to better gut health and symptom management. Remember, your journey to improved digestive health is unique. It may require some experimentation to find the fasting and mindful eating strategies that work best for you. Keep a journal, consult with a healthcare provider, and be patient with yourself along the way.

Chapter 10: Mindful Sleep Practices for Better Health

10.1 The Importance of Quality Sleep

In the hectic day of modern life, sleep is often the first casualty. We proudly wear our exhaustion as a badge of honor, as if sleepless nights are a sign of our dedication and productivity. But the reality is that sleep deprivation has serious health implications, and it's time we recognize the true value of a good night's rest.

Understanding the Health Implications of Sleep Deprivation

Picture this: You're at the wheel, driving down a winding road with your foot on the gas pedal. But instead of a well-rested driver, you're navigating this journey with a fatigued and sleep-deprived version of yourself. The road ahead blurs, your reaction time slows, and the risk of an accident skyrockets. This analogy isn't far from the truth. When you don't get enough sleep, your body and mind are forced to operate in a diminished state, much like that exhausted driver.

Sleep isn't a luxury; it's a biological necessity. Without it, our bodies and minds suffer. Sleep deprivation has been linked to a host of health issues, both physical and mental. For starters, it weakens our immune system, making us more susceptible to illnesses. Your body's ability to fight off infections and heal itself relies on a good night's sleep.

Additionally, sleep deprivation wreaks havoc on our mental health. It's a well-known fact that a sleepless night can leave you feeling irritable and emotionally fragile. But it goes deeper than that. Chronic sleep deprivation is linked to an increased risk of anxiety and depression. It's as if your mind becomes a stormy sea, tossing and turning in the darkness.

The list of health problems associated with inadequate sleep goes on: obesity, diabetes, heart disease, and even a shorter lifespan. It's not an exaggeration to say that quality sleep is the cornerstone of good health.

The Role of Mindful Living in Improving Sleep Quality

So, how do we break free from the cycle of sleep deprivation and reclaim our health and well-being? The answer lies in mindful living. Mindfulness isn't just about meditation and deep breathing exercises. It's a way of life that can extend into every facet of our existence, including our sleep patterns.

Let's start with the concept of mindful awareness. This involves being fully present in the moment, which can be applied to your bedtime routine. When you approach sleep with mindfulness, you're not merely going through the motions; you're consciously engaging in the process. This means setting aside electronic devices, dimming the lights, and creating a calm and soothing atmosphere in your bedroom.

Mindful living also encourages a closer examination of your daily habits. Are you overloading your schedule and sacrificing sleep to meet deadlines or social obligations? Are you consuming caffeine or engaging in stimulating activities too close to bedtime? Mindfulness prompts us to reevaluate these choices and make adjustments that prioritize sleep.

Another aspect of mindful living is stress management. Chronic stress is a notorious sleep thief. When we're consumed by worries and anxieties, it's nearly impossible to slip into a peaceful slumber. Mindfulness techniques, such as progressive muscle relaxation and mindful breathing, can help you unwind and calm your mind before bedtime.

But perhaps one of the most powerful tools in the mindful sleep arsenal is the practice of gratitude. Taking a moment before sleep to reflect on the positive aspects of your day can shift your focus away from stress and anxiety. It can be as simple as acknowledging the comfortable bed you're lying in, the safety of your home, or the loving relationships in your life.

Establishing a Sleep-Friendly Environment
Creating a sleep-friendly environment is an essential component of mindful living. Think of your bedroom as a sanctuary for rest and rejuvenation. It should be a place where your body and mind can unwind, free from distractions and stressors.

Start with your mattress and pillows. Invest in a comfortable and supportive mattress that suits your preferences. Pillows should provide adequate neck and head support, aligning your spine as you sleep. Your goal is to wake up feeling refreshed, not with a sore back or neck.

Now, let's talk about lighting. Our bodies are finely tuned to respond to natural light cycles. During the day, expose yourself to bright natural light to support your circadian rhythm. In the evening, avoid harsh overhead lights. Instead, opt for soft, warm, and dim lighting. Consider using blackout curtains to block out external light sources that can disrupt your sleep.

The temperature in your bedroom matters too. The ideal sleeping temperature is typically cooler than the rest of your home. Most people find a range between 60 to 67 degrees Fahrenheit (15 to 19 degrees Celsius) comfortable for sleep. Experiment with different settings to find what works best for you.

Lastly, minimize noise pollution. Earplugs or white noise machines can be incredibly helpful if you live in a noisy neighborhood or have disruptive environmental sounds. Your goal is to create an oasis of tranquility where your mind can drift into a peaceful slumber.

Quality sleep is not a luxury—it's a vital pillar of health. Mindful living can transform your sleep habits and, in turn, your overall well-being. By understanding the health implications of sleep deprivation, incorporating mindfulness into your sleep routine, and establishing a sleep-friendly environment, you can embark on a journey toward better sleep and better health. Remember, the path to wellness starts with a good night's rest.

10.2 Mindful Sleep Hygiene

In our busy day, a good night's sleep can sometimes feel like an elusive dream. We toss and turn, our minds racing with thoughts of the day that was or the day to come. Sound familiar? You're not alone. Sleep troubles plague millions of people worldwide. Fortunately, the practice of mindfulness can be your secret weapon to reclaiming restful nights and reaping the incredible benefits of rejuvenating sleep.

Mindful Pre-Sleep Rituals for Relaxation

Before diving into mindfulness techniques tailored for better sleep, let's discuss the importance of establishing mindful pre-sleep rituals. These rituals are your gateway to a restful night's sleep. They signal to your body and mind that it's time to wind down, relax, and prepare for slumber.

1: Create a Tranquil Sleep Environment

Your sleep environment plays a crucial role in your ability to relax and drift into a peaceful sleep. Ensure your sleep space is clutter-free, clean, and comfortable. Consider the following:

- Declutter Your Sleep Sanctuary: Remove any distractions or unnecessary items from your bedroom. A cluttered environment can create mental clutter, making it difficult to relax.

- Optimize Your Bedding: Invest in a comfortable mattress and pillows that support your body's natural alignment. Choose soft, breathable bedding that promotes relaxation.

- Control Ambient Light: Dim the lights or use blackout curtains to block out external light sources that may interfere with your sleep.

- Adjust the Temperature: Keep your bedroom at a comfortable temperature, typically on the cooler side, to promote deep sleep.

- Reduce Noise: Minimize noise disruptions by using earplugs or a white noise machine if needed.

2: Establish a Relaxing Pre-Bedtime Routine

A mindful pre-sleep routine is your ticket to unwinding and signaling to your body that it's time to transition into sleep mode. Consider incorporating these relaxation practices into your evening routine:

- Digital Detox: Turn off electronic devices at least an hour before bedtime. The blue light emitted by screens can interfere with the production of melatonin, a hormone that regulates sleep.

- Gentle Stretching or Yoga: Engage in gentle stretching or a short yoga session to release any physical tension accumulated during the day.

- Warm Bath or Shower: A warm bath or shower can relax your muscles and prepare you for sleep. You can even add soothing essential oils like lavender to enhance the relaxation effect.

- Reading or Journaling: Reading a calming book or journaling your thoughts can help you unwind and clear your mind.

- Mindful Breathing: Practice deep, diaphragmatic breathing to calm your nervous system. Inhale deeply through your nose, hold for a few seconds, and exhale slowly through your mouth. Focus on the rise and fall of your breath.

3: The Power of Guided Meditation

Guided meditation is a powerful tool in your pre-sleep toolkit. It helps you shift your focus away from the day's stresses and into a state of relaxation. Here's a simple guided meditation to try before bedtime:

1. Find a Comfortable Position: Sit or lie down in a comfortable position. Close your eyes and take a few deep breaths to settle in.

2. Body Scan: Mentally scan your body from head to toe, noting any areas of tension or discomfort. As you do this, consciously release and relax each area.

3. Focus on Your Breath: Shift your attention to your breath. Notice the sensation of your breath as it enters and leaves your body. Imagine each breath carrying away tension and worry.

4. Visualize a Peaceful Scene: Picture yourself in a tranquil place – it could be a beach, a forest, or a cozy cabin in the mountains. Engage all your senses in this visualization, imagining the sights, sounds, smells, and sensations.

5. Affirmations for Sleep: Repeat a soothing sleep affirmation silently to yourself. For example, "I am safe, and I am at peace. My mind and body are ready for restful sleep."

6. Continue to Breathe: As you maintain your focus on your breath and your chosen scene, allow yourself to drift into a state of deep relaxation. If your mind begins to wander, gently bring your attention back to your breath and the visualization.

7. End with Gratitude: Conclude the meditation by expressing gratitude for the day and the opportunity to rest. Open your eyes slowly, feeling refreshed and ready for a night of rejuvenating sleep.

By incorporating these mindful pre-sleep rituals into your evening routine, you set the stage for a more restful and restorative night's sleep. But what if, despite your best efforts, you still find yourself struggling with insomnia or disrupted sleep patterns? That's where mindfulness techniques for overcoming insomnia come into play.

Mindfulness Techniques for Overcoming Insomnia

Insomnia can be a frustrating and exhausting experience. It often feels like a battle between your desire to sleep and your restless mind. Fortunately, mindfulness offers effective tools to help you break free from the cycle of insomnia.

1: Embrace the Present Moment

Insomnia often stems from ruminating on past events or worrying about the future. Mindfulness encourages you to focus on the here and now. When you find yourself lying awake, shift your attention to your immediate surroundings.

- Grounding Technique: Begin by gently acknowledging the sensation of your body on the bed, the weight of your blankets, and the texture of your pillow. Pay attention to the sounds in your environment, whether it's the hum of a distant car or the rustle of leaves in the wind.

- Observation Without Judgment: As thoughts arise, observe them without judgment. Don't berate yourself for not sleeping or worry about the consequences of a sleepless night. Instead, acknowledge the thoughts and gently let them go, returning your focus to the present moment.

2: Progressive Muscle Relaxation

Progressive muscle relaxation is a technique that can help release physical tension and promote relaxation. Here's how it works:

- Starting at Your Toes: Begin by tensing the muscles in your toes for a few seconds, then release. Move up to your feet, calves, thighs, and so on, progressively working your way through your entire body.

- Deep Breathing: As you tense and release each muscle group, synchronize your breath with the movement. Inhale as you tense the muscles, and exhale as you release.

- Focus on Sensations: Pay close attention to the sensations as you release tension in each muscle group. Visualize the tension melting away, leaving you feeling more relaxed and at ease.

Progressive muscle relaxation can help alleviate physical tension, making it easier for your body to slip into a state of sleep readiness.

3: Mindful Sleep Journaling

Keeping a mindful sleep journal can help you identify patterns and triggers that contribute to your insomnia. Here's how to get started:

- Recording Your Sleep Habits: Each night before bed, jot down your sleep habits. Include the time you went to bed, the time you woke up, and any wakeful periods during the night.

- Emotions and Thoughts: Note any emotions or thoughts that were prevalent before or during sleep. Were you anxious, stressed, or preoccupied with something specific?

- Diet and Activity: Record your dietary choices and physical activities throughout the day. Sometimes, what you consume and how you move can impact your sleep quality.

- Sleep Environment: Evaluate your sleep environment. Did you follow the pre-sleep rituals discussed earlier? Were there any disruptions, such as noise or excessive light?

- Sleep Outcomes: After each night's sleep, record the quality of your sleep and how you felt upon waking. Did you wake up feeling refreshed, or did you experience fatigue and grogginess?

Over time, reviewing your sleep journal can help you identify potential triggers for your insomnia and make informed adjustments to your routine.

Sleep and Its Impact on Disease Prevention
Now that we've explored mindful pre-sleep rituals and techniques for overcoming insomnia, let's delve into the profound impact of sleep on disease prevention. Sleep is not merely a time of rest; it's a vital period during which your body undergoes essential processes that contribute to overall health.

1: The Power of REM Sleep

Rapid Eye Movement (REM) sleep is a crucial phase of the sleep cycle, during which your brain becomes highly active, and vivid dreaming occurs. REM sleep is essential for cognitive function, memory consolidation, and emotional well-being.

- Memory Consolidation: REM sleep plays a vital role in consolidating and organizing memories, making it easier for you to learn and retain information.

- Emotional Processing: During REM sleep, your brain processes and regulates emotions, helping you cope with daily stressors and maintain emotional balance.

- Brain Detoxification: Research suggests that REM sleep facilitates the removal of waste products and toxins from the brain, potentially reducing the risk of neurodegenerative diseases.

2: The Immune System and Sleep

Adequate sleep is a cornerstone of a robust immune system. While you sleep, your body's immune system works diligently to detect and combat pathogens. Sleep deprivation can weaken your immune response, making you more susceptible to infections and illnesses.

- Cytokine Production: Sleep supports the production of cytokines, proteins that regulate inflammation and immune responses. Inadequate sleep can disrupt this delicate balance, contributing to chronic inflammation.

- Immune Memory: Your body forms immune memory during sleep, which helps it recognize and defend against previously encountered pathogens. This is why a good night's sleep can bolster your body's ability to fight off infections.

- Stress Reduction: Quality sleep reduces stress hormone levels, promoting a more harmonious relationship between your immune system and the stress response.

3: Sleep and Chronic Disease Risk

Chronic sleep deprivation has been linked to an increased risk of various chronic diseases, including heart disease, diabetes, obesity, and even cancer. Let's take a closer look at these connections:

- Heart Disease: Poor sleep is associated with hypertension, inflammation, and irregular heartbeat, all of which are risk factors for heart disease.

- Diabetes: Sleep deprivation can disrupt the body's ability to regulate blood sugar, increasing the risk of developing type 2 diabetes.

- Obesity: Lack of sleep affects hunger-regulating hormones, leading to increased appetite and cravings for high-calorie, sugary foods.

- Cancer: Some studies suggest that insufficient sleep may be a contributing factor in the development of certain cancers due to disrupted circadian rhythms.

Understanding the profound impact of sleep on disease prevention underscores the importance of prioritizing quality sleep in your life. The mindful sleep practices and techniques discussed in this chapter are your gateway to achieving that restorative sleep and fortifying your body's defense against illness.

Sleep is not an indulgence; it's a necessity. It's a fundamental component of self-care and disease prevention. By incorporating mindful pre-sleep rituals, overcoming insomnia with mindfulness techniques, and recognizing the far-reaching benefits of restorative sleep, you empower yourself to take control of your health and well-being.

In the fast-paced world we live in, where stress and distractions are abundant, remember this: sleep is your sanctuary. It's where your body and mind rejuvenate, where your cells repair and your spirit finds solace. Embrace the power of mindful sleep practices, and let them guide you to a place of deep and restful slumber, where your health and vitality are nurtured night after night. Sweet dreams.

10.3 Mindful Living Beyond the Bedtime

The benefits of mindfulness extend far beyond just the hours you spend in bed. By cultivating mindfulness during your waking hours, you can set the stage for restful and rejuvenating sleep each night. In this subchapter, we're going to explore how you can incorporate mindfulness into your daytime routines to significantly improve the quality of your sleep.

Incorporating Mindfulness into Daytime Routines for Better Sleep

Have you ever found yourself tossing and turning at night, your mind racing with worries and to-do lists? Many of us experience this, and it can make falling asleep and staying asleep a real challenge. But what if I told you that the quality of your sleep is deeply connected to how you spend your daytime hours?

One of the most effective ways to prepare your mind and body for restful sleep is to practice mindfulness throughout the day. Mindfulness is simply the practice of paying attention to the present moment without judgment. When you're mindful, you're fully engaged in whatever you're doing, whether it's eating, working, or even just walking.

Here are some practical steps to incorporate mindfulness into your daytime routines:

- Mindful Eating: Pay attention to your meals. Taste each bite, savor the flavors, and chew slowly. Avoid distractions like smartphones or television while eating. This practice not only improves digestion but also sets the tone for mindful living.

- Mindful Breathing: Take short breaks throughout the day to focus on your breath. Even just a few minutes of deep, mindful breathing can help you center yourself and reduce stress. It's a simple yet powerful way to stay present.

- Mindful Walking: When you walk, be fully aware of each step. Feel the ground beneath your feet, notice the sensation of movement, and take in your surroundings. Walking mindfully can be incredibly calming and help you clear your mind.

Mindful Stress Management as a Key to Restful Sleep

Stress is one of the most common sleep disruptors. If your mind is racing with worries and anxieties, it's challenging to fall asleep, let alone enjoy a deep and restorative slumber. Fortunately, mindfulness offers a potent antidote to stress.

Mindful living includes a range of stress reduction techniques that you can integrate into your daily life. Here are a few you might find particularly helpful:

- Mindful Meditation: Regular mindfulness meditation practice can be transformative for managing stress. Even just ten minutes of meditation a day can make a significant difference. Find a quiet space, sit comfortably, focus on your breath, and gently bring your attention back when your mind wanders.

- Mindful Body Scanning: This technique involves paying attention to each part of your body, starting from your toes and moving upward. It helps you identify areas of tension and release them, promoting relaxation.

- Mindful Journaling: Write down your thoughts, worries, and emotions in a journal before bedtime. This can help you process your day and clear your mind for sleep.

Success Stories of Individuals Who Transformed Their Sleep with Mindfulness

Let's hear from real people who have experienced remarkable improvements in their sleep quality through the practice of mindfulness.

Success Story 1: Sarah's Journey to Serene Sleep

Sarah, a busy marketing executive, used to struggle with insomnia for years. She felt constantly stressed and found it nearly impossible to unwind at night. Then, she discovered mindfulness.

Sarah incorporated mindfulness into her daily routine, starting with short breathing exercises during her work breaks. She noticed that her stress levels began to decrease, and her mind became more peaceful. Soon, she extended her mindfulness practice to mindful eating and walking.

As the weeks went by, Sarah's sleep improved dramatically. She no longer spent hours lying awake in bed. Instead, she drifted into slumber easily and enjoyed uninterrupted rest. The power of mindfulness had transformed her sleep and, in turn, her overall well-being.

Success Story 2: Mark's Battle with Nightmares

Mark had been plagued by recurring nightmares for as long as he could remember. These nightmares not only robbed him of restful sleep but also left him feeling anxious and drained during the day. Desperate for a solution, he turned to mindfulness.

Mark began practicing mindfulness meditation before bedtime, focusing on calming his mind and releasing fear. Gradually, his nightmares became less frequent, and he started to experience more peaceful nights.

With continued practice, Mark's nightmares ceased altogether. He was finally able to enjoy a peaceful night's sleep, free from the torment of his subconscious mind. Mark's journey demonstrated the profound healing potential of mindfulness for sleep disorders.

Success Story 3: Emily's Battle with Anxiety-Induced Insomnia

Emily, a student facing the pressures of exams and deadlines, suffered from anxiety-induced insomnia. Her racing thoughts prevented her from falling asleep, and she felt exhausted during the day. Mindfulness came to her rescue.

Emily practiced mindfulness during the day, especially when she felt overwhelmed with stress. She learned to observe her anxious thoughts without judgment and gently redirect her focus to the present moment.

Over time, Emily's anxiety lessened, and her sleep improved. She realized that she had the power to calm her mind and relax her body through mindfulness, allowing her to enjoy peaceful nights of sleep, even during the most stressful times of her life.

These stories illustrate that mindfulness is not just a theoretical concept but a practical and transformative tool for enhancing sleep quality. By incorporating mindfulness into your daytime routines and practicing stress-reduction techniques, you too can achieve restful and rejuvenating sleep.

Incorporate these practical steps and take inspiration from these success stories as you embark on your own journey to transform your sleep with mindfulness. Remember, the power to improve your sleep lies within your grasp, and mindfulness is your key to unlock it. Sweet dreams await you as you embrace the practice of mindful living beyond bedtime.

Chapter 11: Mindful and Fasting Lifestyle

11.1 Integrating Mindful Living and Fasting

Welcome to final phase of transformative journey toward a healthier, more vibrant you—a journey that merges the ancient wisdom of mindfulness with the power of fasting. In this subchapter, we'll explore the art of combining mindful living and fasting to create a holistic lifestyle that nurtures your body, mind, and spirit.

Creating a Holistic Lifestyle that Combines Mindfulness and Fasting

Imagine your life as a canvas, waiting for you to paint it with vibrant colors of health, vitality, and purpose. This canvas is your holistic lifestyle, and at its heart lies the fusion of mindfulness and fasting. Let's delve into how you can craft this masterpiece:

1. Embrace Mindful Eating During Fasting: Fasting doesn't mean deprivation; it's an opportunity to savor every bite when you do eat. Practice mindful eating by fully engaging your senses. Pay attention to the textures, flavors, and aromas of your food. This deep connection with your meals not only enhances your fasting experience but also fosters a healthier relationship with food.

2. Schedule Mindful Breaks: In the hustle and bustle of life, it's easy to forget to pause and breathe. Make it a habit to schedule mindful breaks throughout your day. These short moments of stillness can help you remain centered and

reduce stress. You don't need a meditation cushion; just a few conscious breaths will do wonders.

3. Set Clear Fasting Intentions: Whether you're practicing intermittent fasting or extended fasts, start with a clear intention. Why are you fasting? Is it for weight management, disease prevention, or spiritual growth? Knowing your "why" will keep you motivated and focused during fasting periods.

4. Combine Mindfulness and Movement: Physical activity is an integral part of a healthy lifestyle. Integrate mindfulness into your exercise routine by being fully present in your movements. Feel the ground beneath your feet, the air against your skin, and the rhythm of your body. This not only enhances the benefits of exercise but also makes it a joyful experience.

5. Practice Mindful Self-Reflection: Regularly check in with yourself. How are you feeling physically, mentally, and emotionally? Journaling can be a powerful tool for self-reflection. By keeping a record of your experiences, you can identify patterns, celebrate successes, and navigate challenges more effectively.

Overcoming Challenges and Setbacks on the Mindful Living Journey
Life is a journey, and no journey is without its challenges. As you integrate mindful living and fasting into your lifestyle, you may encounter obstacles along the way.

These challenges are not roadblocks but opportunities for growth:

1. Fasting Fatigue: There may be days when fasting feels challenging, especially in the beginning. On such days, remind yourself of your goals and the benefits you've experienced so far. Practice self-compassion and consider modifying your fasting schedule if necessary.

2. Mind Wandering: During mindfulness practices, your mind may wander. This is completely normal. Instead of getting frustrated, gently guide your attention back to the present moment. Over time, this skill will strengthen, and you'll become more adept at maintaining focus.

3. Social Pressure: Social gatherings and peer pressure can be tricky to navigate when fasting or prioritizing mindful choices. Communicate your intentions with friends and family, and seek their support. Remember, your health and well-being matter most.

4. Plateaus: In any transformative journey, you may encounter plateaus where progress seems to stall. It's important to stay patient and persistent. Plateaus are often followed by breakthroughs. Keep your long-term vision in mind and continue with consistency.

Long-Term Benefits of Sustaining Mindful and Fasting Practices

Now, let's look at the long-term rewards of weaving mindful living and fasting into the fabric of your life:

1. Enhanced Physical Health: Over time, the combination of mindfulness and fasting can lead to improved physical health. You'll likely notice better weight management, increased energy levels, and a reduced risk of chronic diseases.

2. Mental Clarity and Emotional Resilience: Consistent mindfulness practice enhances mental clarity and emotional resilience. You'll find it easier to handle stress, anxiety, and negative emotions, leading to a more balanced and harmonious life.

3. Deeper Connection to Your Body: Mindful living fosters a deeper connection to your body. You'll become more attuned to its signals, allowing you to respond to its needs more effectively.

4. Greater Spiritual Awareness: For some, the mindful and fasting lifestyle becomes a spiritual journey. You may experience a heightened sense of purpose, a connection to the universe, or a deeper understanding of your place in the world.

5. Sustainable Habits: By integrating mindfulness and fasting, you're more likely to develop sustainable habits that support your well-being for the long term. These habits become second nature, allowing you to maintain your health effortlessly.

Remember, the journey of mindful living and fasting is not about perfection; it's about progress. Embrace the small victories, learn from the challenges, and keep moving forward on this path to lasting health and wellness. Your holistic lifestyle, filled with mindfulness and fasting, is a masterpiece in the making—unique, personal, and vibrant.

11.2 Case Studies of Matthew Fight Diabetes and Tips for You

Matthew was diagnosed with type 2 diabetes when he was 45 years old. He was overweight and had high cholesterol. He also felt tired and sluggish all the time.

He decided to try fasting to see if it could help him to reduce his reliance on medication. Matthew had heard about the benefits of fasting for people with diabetes, so he decided to give it a try. He started with a 12-hour fast every day. After a few weeks, he increased his fast to 16 hours per day.

After a few months of fasting, he was able to reduce his medication dosage and eventually go off medication altogether. Matthew also started eating a healthier diet and exercising regularly. After a few months, his blood sugar levels were back to normal and he was able to stop taking all medication.

Matthew's Story in More Depth

Matthew's story is a powerful example of how fasting can be used to reverse type 2 diabetes. Matthew was able to reduce his medication dosage and eventually go off medication altogether by fasting for 16 hours per day.

Matthew believes that fasting helped him to reverse his type 2 diabetes in a number of ways. First, fasting helped to reduce inflammation. Inflammation is a major factor in the development and progression of type 2 diabetes. Second, fasting helped to improve insulin sensitivity. Insulin sensitivity is the ability of the body's cells to respond to insulin. When insulin sensitivity is improved, the body can better use the glucose in the bloodstream. This helps to lower blood sugar levels.

How Fasting Can Help to Reverse Type 2 Diabetes

There is a growing body of scientific evidence that suggests that fasting can help to reverse type 2 diabetes. For example, a study published in the journal Cell Metabolism found that fasting can help to improve insulin sensitivity and reduce inflammation in people with type 2 diabetes.

Another study, published in the journal Diabetes, found that fasting can help to reduce blood sugar levels and improve cardiovascular health in people with type 2 diabetes.

Practical Steps for Using Fasting to Reverse Type 2 Diabetes

If you are considering using fasting to reverse type 2 diabetes, it is important to talk to your doctor first. Your doctor can help you to develop a safe and effective fasting plan.

Here are some practical steps that you can follow when using fasting to reverse type 2 diabetes:

* Start slowly. If you are new to fasting, start with a 12-hour fast every day. After a few weeks, you can gradually increase the length of your fasts.

* Listen to your body. If you start to feel lightheaded or dizzy during a fast, break your fast immediately.

* Stay hydrated. It is important to drink plenty of water during a fast.

* Eat a healthy diet. When you are not fasting, eat a healthy diet that is low in processed foods and high in fruits, vegetables, and whole grains.

* Get regular exercise. Exercise is important for people with type 2 diabetes, even if you are fasting.

Fasting can be a powerful tool for reversing type 2 diabetes. If you are considering using fasting to treat your type 2 diabetes, talk to your doctor first. Your doctor can help you to develop a safe and effective fasting plan.

Additional Tips for Using Fasting to Reverse Type 2 Diabetes

Here are some additional tips that may help you to use fasting to reverse type 2 diabetes:

Focus on mindful eating. When you are eating, pay attention to your hunger and fullness cues. Eat slowly and savor your food.

Avoid processed foods. Processed foods are high in unhealthy fats, sugar, and salt. They can also be low in nutrients.

Eat plenty of fruits and vegetables. Fruits and vegetables are low in calories and high in nutrients. They are also a good source of fiber, which can help to regulate blood sugar levels.

Get regular exercise. Exercise helps to improve insulin sensitivity and reduce inflammation.

If you are consistent with fasting and mindful eating, you may be able to reverse your type 2 diabetes and achieve long-term health.

Matthew's Personal Advice

Matthew has some personal advice for people who are considering using fasting to reverse type 2 diabetes:

Be patient and persistent. It takes time to reverse type 2 diabetes. Don't expect to see results overnight.

Listen to your body. If you start to feel lightheaded or dizzy during a fast, break your fast immediately.

Don't be afraid to experiment. There are different types of fasting, so find one that works best for you.

Be kind to yourself. Reversing type 2 diabetes is a journey, not a destination. Be patient with yourself and celebrate your successes along the way.

Matthew add that it is important to have a positive mindset when using fasting to reverse type 2 diabetes. Believe in yourself and in your ability to heal. If you have a positive mindset, you are more likely to be successful.

Matthew also encourage people to talk to their doctor before starting any new fasting regimen. Your doctor can help you to develop a safe and effective fasting plan that is right for you.

11.3 Case Studies of Susan Fight Cancer and Her Personal Advice

Susan was diagnosed with stage IV breast cancer when she was 40 years old. Her doctors told her that her cancer was aggressive and that she had a poor prognosis. They gave her six months to live.

Susan was not ready to give up on her life. She decided to try mindful living and fasting to see if it could help her to heal. She started by reading books and articles about mindful living and fasting. She also started practicing meditation and yoga.

Susan also started fasting. She started with a 12-hour fast every day. After a few weeks, she increased her fast to 16 hours per day.

After a few months of mindful living and fasting, Susan's cancer went into remission. She was able to stop all treatment and she is now cancer-free.

Susan's Story in More Depth

Susan's story is a powerful example of how mindful living and fasting can be used to heal from cancer. Susan was given a poor prognosis, but she refused to give up. She turned to mindful living and fasting, and she was able to achieve remission.

Susan believes that mindful living and fasting helped her to heal in a number of ways. First, mindful living helped her to reduce stress. Stress can weaken the immune system and make it more difficult to heal. Second, fasting helped to reduce inflammation. Inflammation is a major factor in cancer development and progression. Third, fasting helped to boost Susan's immune system. A strong immune system is essential for fighting cancer.

How Mindful Living and Fasting Can Help to Heal Cancer

There is a growing body of scientific evidence that suggests that mindful living and fasting can help to heal cancer. For example, a study published in the journal *Cancer* found that mindfulness meditation can help to reduce stress and improve immune function in people with cancer.

Another study, published in the journal *Autophagy*, found that fasting can help to activate autophagy, a cellular process that helps to remove damaged cells and debris from the body. Autophagy is thought to play a role in cancer prevention and treatment.

Practical Steps for Using Mindful Living and Fasting to Heal Cancer

If you are considering using mindful living and fasting to heal from cancer, it is important to talk to your doctor first. Your doctor can help you to develop a safe and effective plan.

Here are some practical steps that you can follow when using mindful living and fasting to heal cancer:

1. Start slowly. If you are new to mindful living and fasting, start with small changes. For example, you could start by meditating for five minutes each day or fasting for 12 hours once a week.

2. Listen to your body. If you start to feel lightheaded or dizzy during a fast, break your fast immediately.

3. Stay hydrated. It is important to drink plenty of water during a fast.

4. Eat a healthy diet. When you are not fasting, eat a healthy diet that is low in processed foods and high in fruits, vegetables, and whole grains.

5. Get regular exercise. Exercise is important for people with cancer, even if you are fasting.

Mindful living and fasting can be powerful tools for healing from cancer. If you are considering using mindful living and fasting to treat your cancer, talk to your doctor first. Your doctor can help you to develop a safe and effective plan.

Additional Tips for Using Mindful Living and Fasting to Heal Cancer

Here are some additional tips that may help you to use mindful living and fasting to heal cancer:

* Focus on your breath. When you are meditating or fasting, focus on your breath. This can help to reduce stress and anxiety.

* Visualize yourself healing. When you are meditating or fasting, visualize yourself healing from cancer. This can help to boost your immune system and promote healing.

* Be patient and persistent. It takes time to heal from cancer. Be patient and persistent with your mindful living and fasting practice.

Susan's Personal Advice

Susan has some personal advice for people who are considering using mindful living and fasting to heal from cancer:

"Don't give up hope. I was given a poor prognosis, but I refused to give up. I knew that there had to be another way to heal. Mindful living and fasting gave me the hope that I needed to keep going."

"Listen to your body. Pay attention to how you feel when you are meditating and fasting. If you start to feel lightheaded or dizzy, break your fast immediately. It is important to be gentle with yourself."

"Be patient and persistent. It takes time to heal from cancer. Don't expect to see results overnight. Just keep practicing mindful living and fasting, and trust that your body is healing."

Susan's story is an inspiration to us all. She showed us that it is possible to heal from cancer, even when the odds are stacked against us. If you are facing cancer, I encourage you to consider using mindful living and fasting as part of your treatment plan. It may just give you the hope and healing that you need.

Here are some additional tips that may help you to overcome cancer with mindful living and fasting:

Find a support community. There are many online and offline support groups for people with cancer. Talking to other people who are going through the same thing can be very helpful.

Don't be afraid to ask for help. If you are struggling to cope with cancer, don't be afraid to ask for help from your friends, family, or a therapist.

Focus on the present moment. Mindful living can help you to focus on the present moment and appreciate the little things in life. This can be helpful when you are going through a difficult time.

Believe in yourself. You are stronger than you think. Believe in yourself and your ability to heal.

If you are facing cancer, I encourage you to never give up hope. There is always hope for healing. Mindful living and fasting can be powerful tools for overcoming cancer.

Conclusion

Congratulations! You've embarked on a transformative journey through the pages of this book, exploring the profound synergy of mindful living and fasting. As we conclude this adventure, let's reflect on the invaluable wisdom you've gained and the path ahead towards lasting wellness.

Throughout our exploration, you've discovered that this journey is not just about the absence of disease; it's about the presence of vitality, purpose, and profound well-being. It's about embracing a holistic approach to health that nurtures not only your body but also your mind and spirit.

Here are some key takeaways to solidify the wisdom you've acquired and guide you on your ongoing journey:

1. Your Body is a Precious Gift: Your body is not a battleground; it's a sanctuary. Treat it with the utmost care and respect. Nurture it with nourishing foods, movement, and mindfulness. When you approach your body with love and appreciation, it responds with health and vitality.

2. Mindful Living is a Lifelong Practice: Mindfulness is not a destination but a journey. It's a practice you can weave into every aspect of your life. Whether you're eating a meal, taking a walk, or engaging in a conversation, the power of mindfulness is always at your disposal. Continue to deepen your mindfulness practice over time.

3. Fasting is a Tool, Not a Fad: Fasting is a powerful tool in your wellness toolkit. It's not a passing trend but a time-tested practice with profound benefits. Use fasting wisely, guided by your unique needs and goals. Experiment, learn, and adapt as you go. It's not about perfection but progress.

4. Self-Compassion is Essential: Be kind to yourself along this journey. You will face challenges and setbacks, and that's okay. Embrace self-compassion and treat yourself with the same kindness you would offer a friend. Remember, your path to wellness is a marathon, not a sprint.

5. Community and Support Matter: You don't have to walk this path alone. Seek out a community of like-minded individuals who share your passion for mindful living and fasting. Share your experiences, learn from others, and offer support. A supportive community can make all the difference.

6. Celebrate Your Progress: Celebrate every step of your journey, no matter how small. Each positive change, every moment of mindfulness, and every fast completed is a triumph. Celebrate these victories to stay motivated and inspired.

7. Personalize Your Wellness: Your journey is unique, and so are your needs. Embrace personalized wellness by tailoring your mindful living and fasting practices to align with your individual goals, preferences, and circumstances.

8. Embrace the Long-Term Vision: Wellness is not a destination but a lifelong pursuit. Keep your long-term

vision in mind as you make daily choices. Consistency is key, and small, sustainable changes lead to lasting results.

9. Stay Curious and Open-Minded: Wellness is a field that evolves with new discoveries and research. Stay curious, open-minded, and willing to adapt as new insights emerge. Your journey is a dynamic and ever-unfolding one.

10. Share Your Wisdom: As you experience the benefits of mindful living and fasting, consider sharing your wisdom with others. You may become an inspiration and guide for those seeking to transform their lives.

Now, let's talk about your next steps on this remarkable journey:

1. Set Clear Goals: Reflect on your aspirations for wellness. What do you hope to achieve with mindful living and fasting? Write down your goals, and break them into manageable steps.

2. Create a Wellness Plan: Based on your goals, craft a wellness plan that includes mindful living practices, fasting schedules, and other wellness strategies. Make it flexible to adapt to your evolving needs.

3. Stay Accountable: Share your plan with a trusted friend or mentor who can help keep you accountable. Accountability partners can provide motivation and support when you need it most.

4. Continue Learning: Wellness is an ongoing education. Stay informed about the latest research, trends, and best practices in mindful living and fasting. Continue to deepen your knowledge and refine your approach.

5. Prioritize Self-Care: Self-care is not selfish; it's essential. Dedicate time each day for self-care activities that replenish your physical, mental, and emotional well-being.

6. Give Back: Consider sharing your knowledge and experiences with others. Whether through mentoring, writing, or leading workshops, your journey can inspire and help others on their path to wellness.

As we part ways, remember that your journey to wellness is a lifelong adventure, filled with growth, transformation, and boundless potential. Every day is an opportunity to nurture your body, awaken your mind, and nourish your spirit. You have the power to shape your destiny and create a life of vibrant health and vitality.

I leave you with this thought: Wellness is not an achievement; it's a way of living. It's a continuous journey of self-discovery, self-care, and self-empowerment. Embrace it with an open heart and an open mind, and let the beauty of mindful living and fasting enrich every moment of your life.

May your journey be filled with abundance, joy, and radiant well-being. Farewell, dear reader, and may you thrive on your path to wellness.

www.ingramcontent.com/pod-product-compliance
Lightning Source LLC
Chambersburg PA
CBHW070934260726
48661CB00003B/985